Blood Group Systems: Duffy, Kidd and Lutheran

Editors

Steven R. Pierce, SBB(ASCP)
Supervisor, Immunohematology Consultation Laboratory
Community Blood Center of Greater Kansas City
Kansas City, Missouri

Colin R. Macpherson, MD
Medical Director
Hoxworth Blood Center
Cincinnati, Ohio

American Association of Blood Banks
Arlington, Virginia
1988

Mention of specific products or equipment by contributors to this American Association of Blood Banks publication does not represent an endorsement of such products by the American Association of Blood Banks, nor does it necessarily indicate a preference for those products over other similar competitive products.

Efforts are made to have publications of the AABB consistent in regard to acceptable practices. However, as new developments in the practice and technology of blood banking occur, AABB's Committee on Standards recommends changes when indicated from available information. It is not possible to revise each publication at the time each change is adopted. Thus, it is essential that the most recent edition of the *Standards for Blood Banks and Transfusion Services* be used as the ultimate reference in regard to current acceptable practices.

Copyright © 1988 by the American Association of Blood Banks. All rights reserved. No part of this book may be reproduced or transmitted in any form or by any means, electronic or mechanical, including photocopying, recording, or by any information storage and retrieval system, without permission in writing from the Publisher.

American Association of Blood Banks
1117 North 19th Street, Suite 600
Arlington, Virginia 22209

ISBN No. 0-915355-55-8
First Printing
Printed in the United States

Library of Congress Cataloging-in Publication Data

Blood group systems.

   Bibliography: p.
   Includes index.
   1. Blood groups—Duffy system. 2. Blood groups—Kidd system. 3. Blood groups—Lutheran system.
I. Pierce, Steven R. II. Macpherson, Colin.
III. American Association of Blood Banks.
QP98.B543   1988   612'.11825   88-19267
ISBN 0-915355-55-8

Technical/Scientific Workshops Committee

Dennis M. Smith, Jr, MD, Chairman

Michael L. Baldwin, MT(ASCP)SBB
Katherine B. Carlson, MT(ASCP)SBB
Morris R. Dixon, MT(ASCP)SBB
Ronnie J. Garner, MD
Frances L. Gibbs, MT(ASCP)SBB
Sam J. Insalaco, MD
Christina A. Kasprisin, MS, RN
Jerry Kolins, MD
Judith S. Levitt, MT(ASCP)SBB
Colin R. Macpherson, MD
Leo J. McCarthy, MD
Jay E. Menitove, MD
JoAnn M. Moulds, MS, MT(ASCP)SBB
Steven R. Pierce, SBB(ASCP)
Alice R. Barr, SBB(ASCP)
Stephanie H. Summers, MEd, MT(ASCP)SBB
Phyllis Unger, MT(ASCP)SBB
Margaret E. Wallace, MHS, MT(ASCP)SBB
Robert G. Westphal, MD

Contents

Foreword vii

1. **The Duffy Blood Group System: Distribution, Serology and Genetics** 1

   Kathryn M. Beattie, BS, MT(ASCP)SBB

   Characteristics of the Antigens and Antibodies 2
   Distribution of the Duffy Antigens and Phenotypes .. 13
   Genetics 17
   References 20

2. **The Duffy Blood Group System: Biochemistry and Role in Malaria** 27

   Denise A. Valko, MS, MT(ASCP)SBB

   Biochemistry 27
   Duffy and Malaria 31
   Malarial Associations with Other Red Cell Membrane Structures 43
   Development of a Malarial Vaccine 46
   Conclusion 47
   References 47

3. **The Kidd Blood Group System: Serology and Genetics** 53

   Ruth Mougey, MT(ASCP)SBB

   Genetics 53
   Kidd Antigens 57
   Kidd Antibodies 59
   Conclusion 66
   References 66

4. **The Kidd Blood Group System: Drug-Related Antibodies and Biochemistry** 73

   JoAnn Edwards-Moulds, MS, MT(ASCP)SBB

   Chemical and Drug-Related Antibodies 73
   Biochemistry of the Kidd Antigens 77

Disease Association 86
Conclusion 88
References 88

5. **The Lutheran Blood Group System: Serology and Genetics** 93

   Mary N. Crawford, MD

   Common Lutheran Phenotypes and Frequencies 94
   Lutheran Null Phenotypes 96
   High Frequency Lutheran Related Antigens and
      Their Antibodies 100
   Allelic Lutheran Pairs 103
   Lutheran Linkage and Chromosomal Assignment 107
   Lutheran Serology 108
   Clinical Significance of Lutheran and Related
      Antibodies 110
   References 113

6. **The Lutheran Blood Group System: Monoclonal Antibodies, Biochemistry and the Effect of *In(Lu)*** 119

   Geoff Daniels, PhD

   Monoclonal Antibodies 120
   Biochemistry of Lutheran Antigens 122
   Other Antigens Suppressed by *In(Lu)* 127
   The Effect of the Dominant Inhibitor Gene *In(Lu)* 137
   References 140

Index 149

Foreword

This book is the third in a series on the blood group systems. Like its predecessors on ABH/Lewis and Rh, the purpose is to present current understanding of the blood groups, bringing together data that are often fragmented in many publications. In this volume we include three blood group systems: Duffy, Kidd and Lutheran.

The genetics, serology and clinical significance of each system are reviewed and the latest information on biochemistry and disease associations is presented. Included with the Duffy system is a major section on malaria and associated red cell membrane structures. The chapters on the Kidd system emphasize red cell antigen structures and chromosome assignment of the *Jk* genes. In addition to the many Lutheran system antigens and antibodies, non-Lutheran antigens that appear to be influenced by the *In(Lu)* gene are also discussed.

Our appreciation and understanding of the significance of blood groups continues to grow. They are becoming of interest to investigators in fields other than classical blood group serology. We hope this book will prove to be of interest and of value to both our traditional and our newer audiences.

Steven R. Pierce, SBB(ASCP)
Colin R. Macpherson, MD
Editors

In: Pierce, SR, and Macpherson, CR, eds.
Blood Group Systems: Duffy, Kidd and Lutheran
Arlington, VA: American Association
of Blood Banks, 1988

1

The Duffy Blood Group System: Distribution, Serology and Genetics

Kathryn M. Beattie, BS, MT(ASCP)SBB

EARLY IN 1950, THE DISCOVERY of a new blood group system was reported by Cutbush et al.[1] Later that same year Cutbush and Mollison[2] reported more extensively on their findings. The antibody had been found in the serum of a man suffering from hemophilia who had had a number of blood transfusions during the previous 20 years. The antigen was found in 64.9% of 205 blood samples from unrelated persons in the English population. The authors named the system "Duffy" with the permission of the patient in whose serum the antibody had been found. Fy^a was designated as the gene responsible for the antigen, and Fy^b for the allele, which, they were confident, would be discovered later. The following year their confidence was rewarded when anti-Fy^b was found in the serum of a Berlin woman who had had three pregnancies but no transfusions.[3]

In 1955 Sanger et al[4] reported that the most common phenotype in American Blacks is Fy(a−b−) and that it probably represents a product of a silent allele, Fy. Ten years later Chown et al[5] reported a new allele at the *Duffy* locus which they called Fy^x. While many examples of anti-Fy^a and a few of anti-Fy^b were found shortly after the original discoveries, it was 20 years before anti-Fy3 was reported[6] and two more years before anti-Fy4 and anti-Fy5 were described.[7,8]

Studies in 1963 pointed to a probable close linkage between the *Duffy* locus and the locus for congenital zonular cataract.[9] Later work showing linkage between the *Duffy* locus and a structural modification of chromosome 1 established *Duffy*

Kathryn M. Beattie, BS, MT(ASCP)SBB, Director, Reference Laboratory and Technical Education, American Red Cross, Southeastern Michigan Region, Detroit, Michigan as the first human blood group locus to be localized on an autosome.[10]

In 1975 Miller et al[11] reported an association between the Fy^a and Fy^b antigens and invasion of red cells by certain species of malarial parasites.

Anti-Fs has been described.[12] It is thought to be related to the Duffy system.

Finally, a murine monoclonal antibody—designated anti-Fy6—has been reported to recognize an antigen on red cells that is involved in their penetration by some species of *Plasmodium* merozoites.[13]

Characteristics of the Antigens and Antibodies

Anti-Fy^a and Anti-Fy^b

Were it not for the antiglobulin test, the first anti-Fy^a and most examples that have followed would not have been detected. The same is true of other Duffy system antibodies. Only rarely are saline-reactive examples found.[14] Characteristically, the optimum temperature of reactivity is 37 C and activity is enhanced in a low ionic strength medium. Most but not all examples of anti-Fy^a can be detected in low ionic hexadimethrine bromide (Polybrene®) indirect antiglobulin tests.[15] Many of these antibodies activate the complement cascade to bind C3b to antigen-positive red cell membranes. Most are 7S gamma globulins with a molecular weight of 160,000. Hardman and Beck[16] found IgG1 as the only immunoglobulin subclass in 22 of 25 examples of anti-Fy^a and anti-Fy^b. The antibodies are not denatured by 0.1M 2-mercaptoethanol and are stable at 70 C.

Dosage

On titration some examples of anti-Fy^a and anti-Fy^b can discriminate between red cells having a single dose of each antigen and those having two doses. Other techniques based on antibody binding rather than the ability of the antibody to cause agglutination identify dosage more clearly, eg, enzyme-linked immunosorbent assay[17] and fluorescence-activated flow cytometry.[18,19] The sensitivity of these methods is such that even the Fy^{a}Fy^x phenotype can be distinguished from Fy^{x}Fy^x.[17]

Allo- and Autoimmunization

Most Duffy antibodies are the result of alloimmunization by red cells acquired through blood transfusion or transplacental passage. Of interest is a report by Contreras et al[20] of a woman who produced anti-Fy^b as the result of an intrauterine transfusion. She and her husband typed as Fy(a+b−) and the only source of the Fy^b antigen was the blood donor's Fy(a+b+) red cells.

An autoantibody mimicking anti-Fy^b specificity was found in a woman having Fy(a+b−) red cells. By adsorption it was shown that Fy(a+b−) as well as Fy(a−b+) red cells would remove the autoantibody, whereas Fy(a−b−) cells did not. Fy3 and Fy5 specificities were ruled out because the antibody reacted only weakly with enzyme-treated Fy(b+) red cells.[21] An autoantibody mimicking anti-Fy^a has also been described by Mannessier et al.[22]

Frequency and Immunogenicity

Although they may occur singly, most often the Duffy system antibodies are detected in mixtures of other antibodies. Anti-Fy^a occurs somewhat frequently in Caucasians, but anti-Fy^b is relatively rare, being detected only once for every 20 times anti-Fy^a is found. In spite of the fact that the majority of Blacks lack either Fy^a or Fy^b or both, until recently many believed that Blacks did not produce the corresponding antibodies. However, reports from five reference laboratories have made it clear that these antibodies do occur in Blacks, but much less frequently than would be expected from their phenotype as compared with Caucasians.[23-29] In one survey of 110 Duffy antibodies, only 18 were formed by Blacks while 92 were formed by Whites in a patient population having a ratio of 1 Black to 1.7 Whites.[27]

Alloimmunization to Fy^a even in Caucasians is not extremely high, which indicates that these antigens have low immunogenicity. Using data from three series of patients immunized to K and Fy antigens through transfusion or pregnancy,[30] the frequency of Duffy system antibodies was 11.5% (507 antibodies in 4401 patients), compared with 28.5% for anti-K (1254 in 4401 patients). This vast difference in immunogenicity is brought into perspective when one considers that a K+ unit would be represented in only one of 11 donor units while two of three would be Fy(a+). The relative immunization potential of various blood group antigens has been calculated by Giblett[31] by comparing the frequency of the combination of a K-positive donor and K-negative recipient (0.09 × 0.91 = 0.08) with the frequency of an Fy(a+) donor and an Fy(a−) recipient (0.65 × 0.34 = 0.22). Therefore, although the opportunity for immunization to Fy^a is almost three times more frequent than to K, anti-K is observed 2.8 times more often than anti-Fy^a. Thus K is almost nine times more potent as an immunogen than Fy^a.

Fy^a and Fy^b Antigens

Fy^a and Fy^b antigenic determinants are destroyed by proteolytic enzymes such as ficin, papain, bromelin and chymotrypsin, but not by neuraminidase. Fy^a is not affected and Fy^b is only slightly reduced in strength by purified trypsin. "Purified" is stipulated because the trypsin used by blood bankers is usually a crude product that is contaminated with chymotrypsin. The extent of destruction by enzymes is such that treated red cells fail to adsorb their corresponding antibodies, as well as fail to be agglutinated by them. The mode of inactivation of the receptors is not dependent upon the removal of sialic acid and, therefore, is probably the result of proteolytic activity against cell membrane proteins. Red cells from Fy(a−b−) individuals are not sialic-acid-deficient and their electrophoretic mobility is normal.[32] Because of the proteolytic enzyme content of ZZAP reagent[33] and a similar commercial product (W.A.R.M., produced by BCA Organon Teknika Corp, Malvern, PA), Fy^a, Fy^b and Fy6 are destroyed; the antigenic determinants of Fy3, Fy4, Fy5 or Fs are not.

The antigenic determinants are inactivated when the red cells are heated at 56 C for 10 minutes. Formaldehyde also denatures these antigens.[32] These two observations point to the Duffy receptors' being proteins. Additionally, Fy^a and Fy^b antigens are not affected by treatment with 2-aminoethylisothiouronium bromide (AET),[34] but Fy^b may be weakened by 2-hour treatment with chloroquine diphosphate.[35]

Using quantitative immunoferritin microscopy, Masouredis et al[36] determined that red cells having a double dose of Fy^a antigens had 13,300 ± 3500 sites per cell and for Fy^b 13,700 ± 4000. This compared with 6900 ± 610 sites for cells with a single dose of Fy^a or Fy^b antigen.

Although Duffy antigens are not found in various body fluids, red cells stored in a low-pH, low-ionic-strength medium slowly slough antigenic substances into the supernatant. These substances will specifically inhibit anti-Fy^a, anti-Fy^b and anti-Fy3.[37]

Fy^a, Fy^b and Fy3 are not found on leukocytes.[32] Fy^a and Fy^b antigens are also absent from platelets (platelets were not tested for Fy3).[38]

Fy^x, a Weak Variant of Fy^b

In testing 537 families with anti-Fy^a and anti-Fy^b, Chown et al[5] found 20 families with a seeming anomaly of inheritance. In nine, an Fy(a−b+) parent had one or more Fy(a+b−) children. Although the presence of the silent allele Fy might be invoked, it did not account for the fact that in most of these cases the red cells of the apparent Fy(a+b−) parent or child reacted very weakly with some examples of anti-Fy^b. Based on these observations, the investigators thought this was evidence for a new allele to Fy^a, Fy^b and Fy in the Duffy blood group system and designated the product as Fy^x.

Red cells from persons of the Fy^{a}Fy^x phenotype react with selected anti-Fy^b sera by the antiglobulin test, albeit weakly, and they adsorb and elute an antibody with Fy^b specificity. Attempts to separate an antibody specific for Fy^x from anti-Fy^b sera have failed. Thus, perhaps in some respects analogous to D and D^u, the difference between Fy^b and Fy^x is simply quantitative rather than qualitative. The distinction between the products of Fy^x and Fy also depends upon the method and extent of testing, the anti-Fy^b used, and whether serological discrepancies in expected inheritance are investigated.

Fy^xFy^x individuals have been found in northern Sweden and in France.[39, 40] HD50 assays for the Fy^b and Fy3 antigens performed on the red cells from seven Fy^xFy^x, two Fy^bFy^x and four Fy^aFy^x persons led the investigators[40] to conclude that moderate depression of the Fy3 antigen occurs in Fy^aFy^x and Fy^bFy^x individuals and marked depression of Fy3 occurs in Fy^xFy^x persons. Full expression of Fy^b needs normal development of Fy3, in their judgment. The red cells of Fy^xFy^x individuals also appear to react weakly with anti-Fy5[32] and anti-Fy6.[13]

Fy3 and Anti-Fy3

An antibody found in the serum of a Caucasian Australian woman who typed as Fy(a−b−) was named anti-Fy3 by Albrey et al.[6] It reacted with Fy(a+) and Fy(b+) red cells but not with Fy(a−b−) cells. Adsorption-elution studies showed it was not a mixture of anti-Fy^a and anti-Fy^b. This antibody also differed significantly by agglutinating enzyme-treated Fy(a+) or Fy(b+) red cells. These authors speculated that Fy3 might be the precursor for Fy^a and Fy^b, but that has been disputed.

A second example of anti-Fy3 was found along with anti-Fy^a in the serum of a 16-year-old American Black woman during her second pregnancy.[41] She had been transfused with one unit of Fy(a+b+)Fy:3 red cells during her first pregnancy. Her red cells typed as Fy(a−b−)Fy:−3. At the birth of her second child, his red cells were typed as Fy(a−b+)Fy:3 and his direct antiglobulin test was negative.

The third example was found in the serum of an inbred Alberta Cree Indian woman.[42] It is curious that although five of the proposita's children were Fy(a+), she produced anti-Fy3 and not anti-Fy^a. Her mother and a maternal aunt also had Fy(a−b−) red cells and had borne a total of 15 children between them, but neither of them produced Duffy antibodies, indicating that the risk of immunization through pregnancy may be minimal. The proposita's two-unit blood transfusion rather than her nine pregnancies may have been responsible for production of her anti-Fy3.

Surprisingly, several racial differences are apparent in regard to anti-Fy3. First, although the Fy(a−b−) phenotype occurs in 68% of Blacks and an estimated 230,000 annually receive blood transfusions, most of which would be Fy:3 donor units, anti-Fy3 is an uncommon finding among Blacks. Second, when anti-Fy3 has been produced by Blacks, four of four examples were accompanied or preceded by anti-Fy^a.[41,43] Third, others have suggested that anti-Fy3 produced by Blacks is different from that produced by other ethnic groups in being weakly reactive or nonreactive with cord red blood cells in indirect antiglobulin tests[44]; positive results may be obtained by adsorption-elution.[41] Strong reactivity with cord cells was reported with the two antibodies made by Caucasians and one made by a Cree Indian.[6,22,42]

Fy4 and Anti-Fy4

The finding that most Blacks lack Fy^a and Fy^b antigens led to the speculation that Fy(a−b−) represented a null phenotype through inheritance of two silent *Fy* genes. This belief was shaken with the report of an antibody that agglutinated red cells from Blacks but not Whites.[7] The antibody reacted with Fy(a−b−) red cells and with some Fy(a+b−) or Fy(a−b+) cells from Blacks but with none having the Fy(a+b+) phenotype. Despite some variation in the results obtained in three laboratories studying this weak antibody, and the finding that it reacts with protease-treated red cells, the antibody was concluded to be related to the Duffy blood group system. The antibody, named anti-Fy4, was said to detect a product of the *Fy^4* gene. The common Fy(a−b−) phenotype in Blacks might then represent the genotype *Fy^{4}Fy^4* instead of *FyFy*.

While Fy(a+b−) and Fy(a−b+) phenotypes ordinarily indicate double antigen doses in Caucasians, these phenotypes in Blacks would be mainly products of $Fy^a Fy^4$ and $Fy^b Fy^4$, respectively. Only rarely, due to the relatively low frequency of the Fy^a and Fy^b genes, would the phenotypes represent the homozygous condition in Blacks.

While some evidence suggests that Fy^4 is an allele to Fy^a and Fy^b, it may be an allele to Fy^3. The adjudication of which relationship prevails depends upon finding a reliable example of anti-Fy4 and using it to test Black families that have the Fy(a−b−), Fy(a+b−) and Fy(a−b+) phenotypes and being able to account for all Duffy genes, including Fy. Having such a serum would also allow it to be used by flow cytometry to determine dosage in Fy(a−b−) red cell samples and thereby to predict the zygosity of the person.

On the basis of similarity in serological behavior, anti-Fy4 is more like anti-Fy3 than anti-Fy^a or anti-Fy^b. The former antibodies are reactive with enzyme-treated red cells while the latter two are not.

Fy5 and Anti-Fy5

An antibody found in the serum of an 11-year-old American boy of Black ancestry was initially thought to be a further example of anti-Fy3.[8] The child's red cells typed as Fy(a−b−) and his serum agglutinated Fy(a+) or Fy(b+) red cells but not Fy(a−b−) cells from other Blacks. His antibody, however, differed from anti-Fy3 in that it did not react with Rh$_{null}$ red cells despite their being either Fy(a+) or Fy(b+); D−− red cells reacted weakly. Furthermore, unlike anti-Fy3, it agglutinated the Fy(a−b−) red cells of the Caucasian woman who had made anti-Fy3. Apart from Rh and Fy, the antibody showed no interrelationships with other blood group systems.

The authors named the antibody anti-Fy5 and designated the antigen Fy5. Since the maker of the antibody had red cells that lacked Fy5 but had normal Rh antigens, Fy5 could not be a common precursor for both Fy and Rh. They proposed that synthesis of the Fy5 antigen arises by interaction of Rh and $Duffy$ gene products.

A second example was reported 3 years later among a mixture of antibodies in the serum of a multiply transfused American Black woman suffering from sickle cell anemia.[45] After isolation, the antibody reacted in the same fashion as the first one, but the investigators now had the opportunity to test ther the amorphic nor the regulator type was reactive with the anti-Fy5. This led the authors to state: "If interaction between Rhesus and Duffy gene products is necessary for Fy5 antigen synthesis, it must be the *Rh* gene itself and not the X^1r modifier that is involved."

A third example of anti-Fy5 (erroneously called the second example) was also found in the serum of a sickle cell anemia patient among a mixture of other antibodies.[46] The author described a serious delayed transfusion reaction and attributed it to anti-Fy5, but failed to prove that this was the cause, since anti-C and anti-E were also eluted from the patient's posttransfusion red cells.

Anti-Fs

Anti-D, anti-V and another antibody were found in the serum of a Brazilian Black woman whose red cells typed as Fy(a+b+)Fy:3,5. She had had three pregnancies and many blood transfusions.[12] After separation from the others, the third antibody reacted by antiglobulin tests with 79% of Fy(a−b−) red cell samples and with about 14% of Fy(a+b−), Fy(a−b+) and Fy(a+b+) samples from either White or Black donors. The significantly higher frequency of reactions with Fy(a−b−) red cells than with other Duffy phenotypes indicated that anti-Fs was not directed at an unrelated high incidence antigen found in Blacks.

It did not bind complement. The strength of the antibody was low; agglutination ranged from microscopic (score 2 or 3) to reactions barely recognizable macroscopically (score 5 to 7). The weakest reactions were not consistently reproducible, forcing the investigators to establish a cutoff whereby cell samples scoring 5 or more were considered positive while samples scoring less than 5 were called negative. Using these admittedly arbitrary criteria, tests with the serum indicated a clear preference for red cells of the Fy(a−b−) phenotype.

The antibody, which the authors named anti-Fs, differed from anti-Fy4 in that anti-Fs reacted with Fy(a+b+) red cells whereas anti-Fy4 did not. Anti-Fs reactivity was enhanced in tests with papain-treated cells. It was determined to be monospecific and to be a polyclonal protein mainly of an IgG2 subtype, but with lesser amounts of IgG1 and IgG4. Tests for leukocyte antibodies using agglutination and lymphocytotoxicity methods were negative.

Tests indicated that the Fs antigen is present on the red cells of both Black and White newborn infants. This first example of anti-Fs did not cause hemolytic disease of the newborn, and the investigators speculated that other examples having similar serological characteristics would also be unlikely to do so.

Definitive family studies could not be done because of the weakness of the antibody. The limited studies, however, showed that Fs-positive children may be born to Fs-negative parents. The authors stated: "If Fs is inherited as a simple Mendelian characteristic, the controlling gene segregates independently of the *Duffy* genes."

Anti-Fy6 and Fy6

The interest generated by the demonstration that Fy(a−b−) erythrocytes resist the penetration of certain *Plasmodium* merozoites (see Chapter 2) led Nichols et al[13] to search for an alloantibody that might identify the specific Duffy receptor responsible. A murine monoclonal antibody was prepared that reacted with all human red cells except for those of the Fy(a−b−) phenotype. The antibody's positive reactions with Rh_{null} red cells of both the regulator and amorphic types distinguished it from anti-Fy5. With untreated red cells, the antibody reacted in the same fashion as anti-Fy3. However, enzyme treatment of the cells showed a clear distinction. The reactivity of Fy6, like Fy^a and Fy^b antigens, is destroyed by ficin, papain and chymotrypsin in contrast to Fy3 which is enhanced. Trypsin enhances both Fy3 and Fy6.

The mean number of antigenic determinant sites on Fy6 red cells was determined to be 12,200 ± 1260 per cell,[13] closely approximating the 13,300 Fy^a sites.[40] While the investigators saw no visible heterogeneity of binding, they did not test cells from persons known to be heterozygous for Fy6. The Fy6 protein, like Fy^a and Fy^b, appears to have a molecular mass of 46 kilodaltons.

Tests of red cells from nonhuman primates demonstrated that some but not all had the Fy6 epitope. Its presence correlated with susceptibility of the animal's red cells to penetration by the merozoites of *Plasmodium vivax* (see Chapter 2).

Nomenclature

Table 1-1 summarizes the Duffy system antibodies, and Table 1-2 summarizes their reactions with various red cell phenotypes. The nomenclature for the Duffy system for the known alleles is Fy^a and Fy^b or Fy^1 and Fy^2, respectively, in the numerical terminology. Their gene products (antigens) are Fy^a and

Table 1-1. Characteristics of Duffy System Antibodies

Antibody Specificity	Typical Serological Reactivity*								Ability to Bind Complement	Implicated in	
	Saline			LISS or Albumin			Enzyme			HTR†	HDN‡
	22 C	37 C	AGT	22 C	37 C	AGT	37 C	AGT			
Anti-Fyᵃ	rare	rare	yes	rare	rare	yes	no	no	many examples	yes	yes
Anti-Fyᵇ	rare	rare	yes	rare	rare	yes	no	no	many examples	yes	yes
Anti-Fy3	weak	weak	yes	no	no	yes	yes	yes			yes
Anti-Fy4	no	no	yes			yes		yes			
Anti-Fy5	no	no	yes			yes		yes			
Anti-Fy6	no	no	yes			yes	no	no			
Anti-Fs	no	no	yes			yes		yes	no	no	no

*with antigen in commonly used tube techniques
†Hemolytic transfusion reactions
‡Hemolytic disease of the newborn

Table 1-2. Reactions of Duffy System Antibodies with Red Cells of Various Phenotypes

Race of Donor	Red Cell Phenotype	Fy^{a*}	Fy^{b*}	Fy3	Anti-Fy4	Fy5	Fy6*	Fs
Caucasian	Fy(a+b−)	+	0	+	0	+	+	14%+
Caucasian	Fy(a−b+)	0	+	+	0	+	+	14%+
Caucasian	Fy(a+b+)	+	+	+	0	+	+	14%+
Caucasian	Fy(a+b−), D−−	+	0	+	0	+^{w}		NT
Caucasian	Fy(a+b+), Rh$_{null}$ (regulator type)	+	+	+	0	0	+	NT
Caucasian	Fy(a−b+), Rh$_{null}$ (amorphic type)	0	+	+	NT	0	+	NT
Caucasian	Fy(a−b^w+) *Fy^{x}Fy^x* genotype	0	+^{w}	+^{w}	NT	+^{w}	+^{w}	NT
Caucasian	Fy(a−b−) producer of anti-Fy3	0	0	0	+^{w}	+	0	+
Cree Indian	Fy(a−b−) producer of anti-Fy3	0	0	0	+†		NT	NT
Black	Fy(a−b−)	0	0	0	most +	0	0	79%+
Black	Fy(a+b+)	+	+	+	0	+	+	15%+
Black	Fy(a+b−)	+	0	+	most +	+	+	15%+
Black	Fy(a−b+)	0	+	+	most +	+	+	15%+
Black	Fy(a+) or Fy(b+) cord blood	+	+	+^{w}	NT	+	+‡	+§

NT = not tested
*negative reactions are obtained with these antisera when antigen-positive red cells are enzyme treated
† test could not be properly controlled[42]
‡ same strength as adult red cells (Nichols ME, personal communication)
§ same strength as adult red cells

Table 1-3. Examples of Duffy System Notation

Gene	Antigen	Antibody	Phenotypes Positive	Phenotypes Negative
Fy^3	Fy3	anti-Fy3	Fy:3	Fy:$-$3
Fy^4	Fy4	anti-Fy4	Fy:4	Fy:$-$4

Fy^b or Fy1 and Fy2. The antibodies are anti-Fy^a (or anti-Fy1) and anti-Fy^b (or anti-Fy2). Although Fy^x and Fy are genes, no anti-Fy^x or anti-Fy exists. The gene product for Fy^x is a weak Fy^b antigen named Fy^x. The Fy gene has no known product. When this gene occurs in Whites or Orientals, it is usually silent. However, in American Blacks, while Fy can act as a silent gene, phenotypes showing a lack of Fy^a or Fy^b antigens usually have Fy4.

Examples of written notation for the Duffy system are shown in Table 1-3. A written phenotype expresses the actual results of testing. For example, the common phenotype of red cells from an American Black person tested with anti-Fy^a, anti-Fy^b, anti-Fy3, anti-Fy4, anti-Fy5 and anti-Fy6 might be written: Fy(a$-$b$-$)Fy:$-$3,4,$-$5,$-$6. A typical phenotype for the cells of a Caucasian donor typed with the same reagents could be: Fy(a+b$-$)Fy:3,$-$4,5,6.

Clinical Significance of Duffy Antibodies

Although anti-Fy^a has often been cited as a cause of hemolytic transfusion reactions,[47] only seven reactions (four immediate, three delayed, none fatal) were seen at the Mayo Clinic among 268,000 transfusions given in the 10-year period 1964-1973.[48] A few fatal transfusion reactions have also been reported.[49,50]

Inasmuch as anti-Fy^b occurs much less frequently, the paucity of reports of transfusion reactions is not unexpected. However scarce, anti-Fy^b has caused delayed reactions[51] and deaths.[52]

Anti-Fy3 and anti-Fy4 have not been implicated in transfusion reactions. Anti-Fy5 has been incriminated, but the anti-C and anti-E in the patient's serum may have been equally culpable.[46]

The role of the Fy^a antigen in kidney transplantation was examined when a kidney from an Fy(a+) sibling was transplanted to a patient who had an anti-Fy^a titer of 16. Three days after the transplant, the titer rose to 64, but decreased to 32 by the eighth day and remained at that level through the 44th day in spite of an acute rejection episode which was successfully controlled. The authors concluded that Fy^a is not a transplantation antigen.[53]

Anti-Fy^a is not a frequent cause of hemolytic disease of the newborn (HDN) in spite of the antibody's usually being an IgG1 capable of traversing the placenta and in spite of the Fy^a antigen's being well developed early in fetal life. Most reports of HDN due to anti-Fy^a indicate that the infants are not severely affected; however, some have required exchange transfusion.[54] Greenwalt et al[55] in presenting information on 11 cases of HDN involving anti-Fy^a pointed out that five of the mothers had been immunized by transfusions of Fy(a+) blood. Two of the infants in that series died. Phototherapy and two red cell transfusions sufficed as treatment in the only recorded case of an infant affected by HDN due to anti-Fy^b.[56]

Mild HDN affected the third child of the Australian Caucasian woman[6] and the ninth child of the Alberta Cree Indian woman[42] who produced the first and third examples of anti-Fy3, respectively. The newborn son of the young American Black woman who made the second example of anti-Fy3 was unaffected. HDN implicating anti-Fy4 and anti-Fy5 has not been described.

Distribution of the Duffy Antigens and Phenotypes

The Duffy system is remarkable because of the wide divergence in distribution of the antigens among various racial groups. The frequency of Fy^a varies from almost 100% in Melanesians[57] to a very low percentage in African Blacks.[58,59] About two thirds of European and North American Caucasians are Fy(a+).[60] The distribution of Fy^b is equally discriminating. While the Fy^b phenotype is exhibited in over 80% of White populations, it is much less frequent in South African Blacks[57-59] and Asians.[57,61,62] (See Table 1-4.)

The Fy(a−b−) phenotype found in over two thirds of American Blacks varies between 90 and almost 100% in African Blacks.[57,59] On the basis of skin color one might expect Australian aborigines to show similar frequencies for this pheno-

14 BLOOD GROUP SYSTEMS: DUFFY, KIDD AND LUTHERAN

Table 1-4. Racial Distribution of Fy Phenotypes (in Percent)

	Fy(a+b−)	Fy(a−b+)*	Fy(a+b+)	Fy(a−b−)	Fy(a+b+w)†	Fy(a−b+w)‡
Asian						
Chinese§	90.8	0.3	8.9	0		
Japanese[61]	81.5	0.9	17.5	0		
Thai[62]	69	3	28	0		
Australian						
Aborigine[63]	93	0.1	7	0		
Black						
S. African[59]	6	6	0.2	88		
American[4]	9	22	2	68		
Caucasian[60]	18	33	48	0	1.3	0.02

*Fy(a−b+) includes the products of Fy^bFy^b, Fy^bFy^x and Fy^bFy
†Fy(b+w) is the product of the Fy^x gene
‡includes the products of Fy^xFy^x and Fy^xFy
§frequencies observed by M. Lin-Chu, MD, personal communication

type; on the contrary, Fy(a−b−) does not occur. Instead, the frequency of Fy(a+) ranges from 90 to 100%, probably reflecting their Asian antecedents.[63]

The Fy(a−b−) phenotype does exist in other ethnic groups due to the introduction of genes from other races. Sandler et al[64], investigating the origin of sickle cell hemoglobin (HbS) in two groups of native White Sicilians, found blood group evidence of African admixture, including the Fy(a−b−) phenotype in 11% of unrelated individuals and members of families with known HbS. The Fy(a−b−) phenotype has also been found in Moslem, Christian and Druze Arabs and Jewish immigrants from Yemen and Iraq, but not in Sephardi or Ashkenazi Jews.[65]

From the foregoing observations, it is apparent that the incidence of the Fy^a gene is very high in all native Asians, of moderate proportion in Caucasians and relatively low in native Africans. The frequency of the Fy^b gene, as can be seen in Table 1-5, is slightly higher than Fy^a in Caucasians, but as expected, is quite low in Australian aborigines and South African Blacks. The Fy gene occurs in Caucasians but with a frequency of less than 0.001. The frequency of individuals homozygous for the Fy gene ($FyFy$) must be much less than 0.001 inasmuch as no Fy(a−b−) blood samples were found in testing 9617 Whites.[5, 6, 63] Conversely, the incidence of Fy reaches 100% in some African tribes.[13]

Development of Fy Antigens on Fetal Red Cells

Fy^a and Fy^b antigens are well developed at birth[2, 66] and readily detectable early in intrauterine life.[66] Fy^a was found in a fetus of 6 weeks' gestation (20-mm crown-to-heel length) and Fy^b in one of 6-1/2 weeks.[66] Adult strength of the antigens was observed starting at the 12th week of gestation.

Although there is no information on Fy4, both Fy3 and Fy5 are developed at birth but may give weaker reactions than adult cells with some examples of anti-Fy3 or anti-Fy5.[6, 8, 41, 44, 66] The strength of the Fy3 antigen seems to increase shortly after birth as shown by the results of tests on the red cells of one 2-1/2-month-old and one 5-month-old infant.[66]

Fs, an antigenic determinant possibly related to the Duffy blood groups, has been detected on red cells from Black and White newborns.[12]

Duffy Antigens in Other Primate Species

Typing of 12 chimpanzees showed that the red cells of 11 had the phenotype Fy(a−b+)Fy:3 and one had Fy(a−b−)Fy:−3, resulting in approximate gene frequencies of Fy^a 0.00, Fy^b 0.70

Table 1-5. Racial Distribution of *Fy* Genes and Genotypes

	Genes				Genotypes								
	Fy^a	*Fy^b*	*Fy^x*	*Fy*	*Fy^aFy^a*	*Fy^aFy^b*	*Fy^bFy^b*	*Fy^aFy*	*Fy^bFy*	*FyFy*	*Fy^aFy^x*	*Fy^bFy^x*	*Fy^xFy*
Asian													
Chinese*	0.945	0.047			0.8930	0.0888	0.0022						
Japanese[61]	0.903	0.097			0.8150	0.1755	0.0094						
Thai[62]	0.8289	0.1711			0.6871	0.2836	0.0293						
Australian													
Aborigine[63]	0.964	0.0360		0.000	0.9293	0.0694	0.0013			0.000			
Black													
S. African[59]	0.0314	0.0302		0.9384	0.00098	0.0019	0.00091	0.0589	0.0567	0.8806			
American[4]	0.0534	0.1220		0.8246	0.0029	0.0130	0.0149	0.0881	0.2012	0.6799			
Caucasian[60]	0.424	0.560	0.015	0.001	0.1798	0.4749	0.3136	<0.0001	0.0127	0.0168	0.0002	0.0001	

*M. Lin Chu, MD, personal communication

and Fy 0.30.[13, 32, 67] A further trip down the evolutionary tree (with one, two or three examples of each species) disclosed that the only gorilla tested[32, 67] had Fy3, weak Fy^b and Fy6 antigens but no Fy^a antigen; none of the other primates had Fy^a, but two *Macacus fascicularis* monkeys had Fy3 and weak Fy^b antigens, the latter detectable only by absorption-elution. Two *M. rhesus* monkeys and two marmosets were Fy(a−b−)Fy:3, but two tree shrews, also negative for both Fy^a and Fy^b, were only weakly positive for Fy3. Two of the New World monkeys (douroucouli and squirrel), but none of the Old World monkeys, had Fy6. Lower in the primates, the red cells of two slow lorises and one bush baby reacted with neither anti-Fy3 nor anti-Fy^b.[32] This evidence suggests that Fy3 must have been an earlier evolutionary development than Fy^b, while Fy^a arose during human ontogeny.

Genetics of the System

Gene Localization and Linkage

The Fy locus,[10] like Rh,[68] is located on chromosome 1. These genes are not linked, but are said to be syntenic—that is, both reside on the same chromosome. While Rh is near the tip of the short arm and Fy is near the centromere, there is controversy about whether Fy is on the short (p) or long (q) arm in the p21 → q23 area of the chromosome. The most recent human gene map[69] indicates that Rh is located 38.9 centimorgans (cM) from the terminus of the short arm of chromosome 1, the red cell enzymes PGD at 18.3, PGM^1 at 71.1 and Fy at 120.5 cM. Considerable other genetic evidence places the Fy site on the long arm of chromosome 1[70-72] and shows linkage of the Fy gene and the genes for antithrombin III[72] and the type 1 hereditary motor and sensory neuropathy.[71]

Inheritance and Synthesis of Duffy Antigens

Fy^a, Fy^b, Fy^x and Fy are alleles—the other Duffy antigens are not produced by alleles at that locus. It is conceivable that the Fy3 antigen might be an interaction product of the Fy^a, Fy^b and Fy^x genes. Fy^3 cannot be an allele at the same locus since red cells of some people are Fy(a+b+) and Fy:3. If Fy^3 is located at a different locus, Fy^4 might be an allele to it since most Blacks who have the Fy(a−b−)Fy:−3 phenotype are Fy:4. Conversely, no Fy(a+b+)Fy:3 red cells are Fy:4. It has been hypothesized that the Duffy system may be comprised of two closely-linked genes at adjacent loci with Fy^a, Fy^b, Fy^x or Fy at one locus and Fy^3 or its allele Fy^4 at a nearby site.[7] In Whites, Fy^a or Fy^b would be at one locus and Fy^3 at the other locus. (See Fig 1-1A.) In Blacks, the most common haplotype would contain Fy and Fy^4. (See Fig 1-1B.)

Fy, a silent gene at the Duffy locus, is an allele of Fy^a, Fy^b and Fy^x. It produces no product and results in the Fy(a−b−) phenotype. Whites with this phenotype are also Fy:−3 but may not have the Fy4 antigen, in contrast to Blacks who usually do have Fy4 in double dose. (See Fig 1-1C.) The observation that the rare Whites having the Fy(a−b−) phenotype have produced anti-Fy3, while Blacks usually do not, points to a different genetic basis for the inheritance of Fy in the two races.[73] That is not to say that the type of Fy transmission seen in Caucasians is limited to that race. It is not, as evidenced by the Cree Indian woman[42] who was Fy(a−b−) Fy:−3 and made anti-Fy3.

The rare Fy(a−b−) phenotype in Whites simply cannot arise through the homozygous inheritance of a suppressor gene independent of Fy. This is ruled out by the failure to find Fy(a+b+) children from matings of Fy(a−b−)Fy:−3 individuals with Fy(a+) or Fy(b+) spouses.

An operator gene at another locus can be invoked to explain the dampening effect on an Fy^b gene and a partner Fy^3 gene to produce the weak expression of Fy^b and Fy3 antigens seen in the Fy^x phenotype.

Whether there are genes such as Fy^5, Fy^6 and Fs is speculative. Because antibodies have been found that recognize epitopes which have been named Fy3, Fy4, Fy5, Fy6 and Fs does not necessarily mean that there are separate genes for each of these products. Nature tends to conserve. Genes may be responsible for multiple products by interaction with other genes, eg, the Le gene which gives rise to both Le^a and Le^b antigens. The serological similarities of anti-Fy3, anti-Fy5 and anti-Fy6 are such that one gene—Fy^3—could be responsible for the total product. The expression of Fy5 depends upon the interaction of a normal Rh gene with a Duffy gene. That Duffy gene could be Fy^3. The Fy3 protein may consist of a protease-resistant area and a protease-sensitive portion— the latter representing the Fy6 epitope. Other speculative genetic pathways for the biosynthesis of some of the Duffy system antigens and hypotheses to explain the phenotypes may be found elsewhere.[74,75]

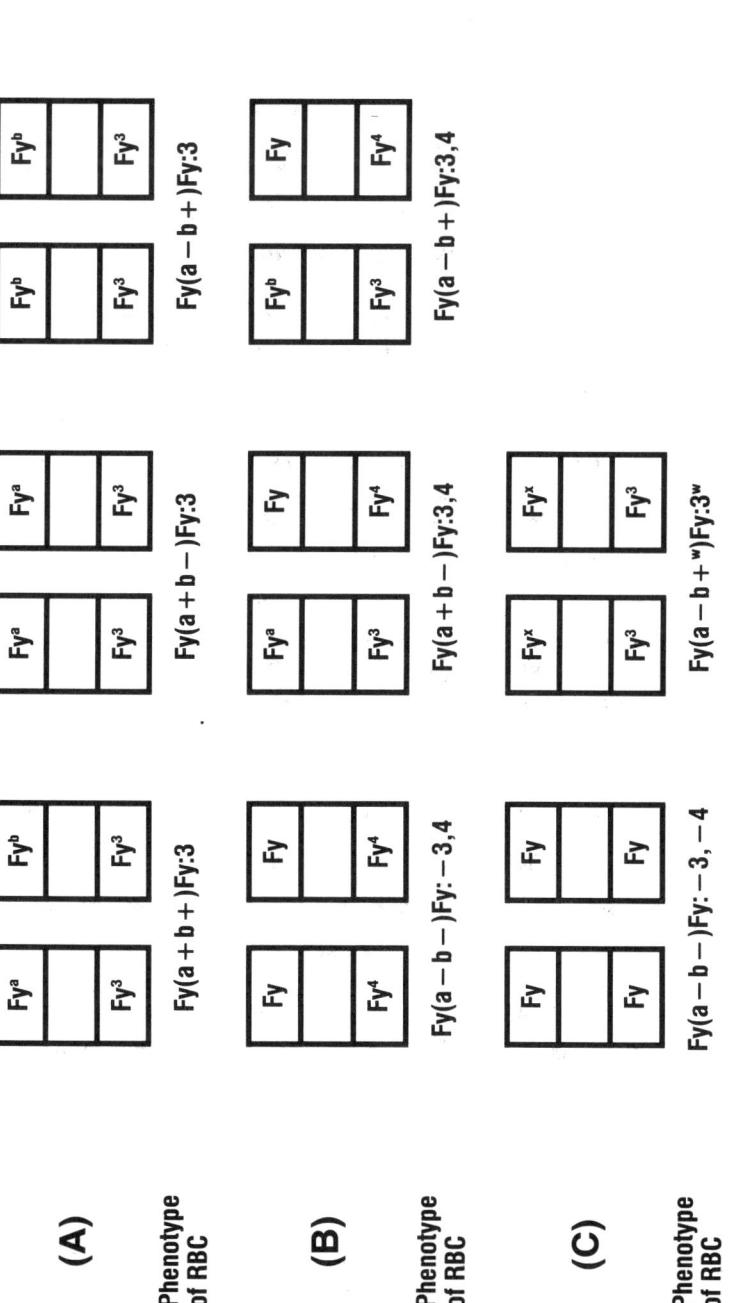

Figure 1-1. (A) Common Duffy system haplotypes in Caucasians, (B) common Duffy system haplotypes in American Blacks and (C) rare Duffy system haplotypes in Caucasians.

References

1. Cutbush M, Mollison PL, Parkin DM. A new human blood group. Nature 1950;165:188-9.
2. Cutbush M, Mollison PL. The Duffy blood group system. Heredity 1950;4:383-9.
3. Ikin EW, Mourant AE, Pettenkofer HJ, Blumenthal G. Discovery of the expected haemagglutinin, anti-Fy^b. Nature 1951;168:1077-8.
4. Sanger R, Race RR, Jack JA. The Duffy blood groups of New York Negroes. The phenotype Fy(a−b−). Br J Haematol 1955;1:370-4.
5. Chown B, Lewis M, Kaita H. The Duffy blood group system in Caucasians: evidence for a new allele. Am J Hum Genet 1965;17:384-9.
6. Albrey JA, Vincent EER, Hutchinson J, et al. A new antibody, anti-Fy3, in the Duffy blood group system. Vox Sang 1971;20:29-35.
7. Behzad O, Lee CL, Gavin J, Marsh WL. A new anti-erythrocyte antibody in the Duffy system: anti-Fy4. Vox Sang 1973;24:337-42.
8. Colledge KI, Pezzulich M, Marsh WL. Anti-Fy5, an antibody disclosing a probable association between the Rhesus and Duffy blood group genes. Vox Sang 1973;24:193-9.
9. Renwick JH, Lawler SD. Probable linkage between a congenital cataract locus and the Duffy blood group locus. Ann Hum Genet 1963;27:67-84.
10. Donahue RP, Bias WB, Renwick JH, McKusick VA. Probable assignment of the Duffy blood group locus to chromosome 1 in man. Proc Nat Acad Sci USA 1968;61:949-55.
11. Miller LH, Mason SJ, Dvorak JA, McGinniss MH, Rothman IK. Erythrocyte receptors for (*Plasmodium knowlesi*) malaria: Duffy blood group determinants. Science 1975;189:561-3.
12. Palatnik M, Junqueira PC, Alves ZMS. Fs: an antigenic determinant possibly related to the Duffy blood group. Rev Fr Transfus Immunohematol 1982;6:629-37.
13. Nichols ME, Rubinstein P, Barnwell J, Rodriguez de Cordoba S, Rosenfield RE. A new human Duffy blood group specificity defined by a murine monoclonal antibody. J Exp Med 1987;166:776-85.
14. Race RR, Sanger R, Lehane D. Quantitative aspects of the blood group antigen Fy^a. Ann Eugen 1955;17:255-66.

15. Letendre PL, William MA, Ferguson, DJ. Comparison of a commercial hexadimethrine bromide method and low-ionic-strength solution for antibody detection with special reference to anti-K. Transfusion 1987;27:138-41.
16. Hardman JT, Beck ML. Hemagglutination in capillaries: correlation with blood group specificity and IgG subclass. Transfusion 1981;21:343-6.
17. Caren LD, Bellavance R, Grumet FC. Demonstration of gene dosage effects on antigens in the Duffy, Ss, and Rh systems using an enzyme-linked immunosorbent assay. Transfusion 1982;22:475-8.
18. Oien L, Nance S, Garratty G. Zygosity determinations using flow cytometry—a superior method (abstract). Transfusion 1985;25:474.
19. Oien LS. Antigen zygosity determinations using flow cytofluorometry. In: Five best essays. 1985 American Association of Blood Banks scholarship awards. Deerfield, IL: Fenwal Laboratories, 1985.
20. Contreras M, Gordon H, Tidmarsh E. A proven case of maternal alloimmunization due to Duffy antigens in donor blood used for intrauterine transfusion. Br J Haematol 1983;53:355-6.
21. van't Veer MB, van Leeuwen I, Haas FJLM, Smelt M, Overbeeke MAM, Engelfriet CP. Red cell auto-antibodies mimicking anti-Fy^b specificity. Vox Sang 1984;47:88-91.
22. Mannessier L, Habibi B, Salmon C. Un nouvel example anti-Fy3 comportant une réactivité pseudo-anti-Fy^a. Rev Fr Transfus Immunohematol 1979;22:195 (in French) cited in Issitt PD. Applied blood group serology. 3rd ed. Miami: Montgomery Scientific, 1985.
23. Kosanke J. Production of anti-Fy^a in Black Fy(a−b−) individuals. Red Cell Free Press 1983;8(3):4.
24. Beattie, KM. Production of anti-Fy^a in Black Fy(a−b−) individuals (letter). Red Cell Free Press 1983;8(3):13.
25. Vengelen-Tyler V. Production of anti-Fy^a in Black Fy(a−b−) individuals (letter). Red Cell Free Press 1983;8(3):14.
26. Issitt PD. Production of anti-Fy^a in Black Fy(a−b−) individuals (letter). Immunohematology 1984;1:11-13.
27. Beattie KM. Production of anti-Fy^a in Black Fy(a−b−) individuals (letter). Immunohematology 1984;1:14.
28. Sosler SD, Saporito C, Fong K, Perkins JT. The relative prevalence of Duffy antibodies in a population of known racial makeup (abstract). Transfusion 1986;26:546.

29. Baldwin M, Shirey RS, Coyle K, Kickler TS, Ness PM. The incidence of anti-Fy^a and anti-Fy^b antibodies in Black and White patients (abstract). Transfusion 1986;26:546.
30. Mollison PL. Blood transfusion in clinical medicine. 7th ed. Oxford: Blackwell Scientific, 1983.
31. Giblett ER. A critique of the theoretical hazard of inter- vs intra-racial transfusion. Transfusion 1961;1:233-8.
32. Marsh WL. Present status of the Duffy blood group system. CRC Crit Rev Clin Lab Sci 1975;5:387-412.
33. Branch DR, Petz LD. A new reagent (ZZAP) having multiple applications in immunohematology. Am J Clin Pathol 1982;78:161-7.
34. Advani H, Zamor J, Judd WJ, Johnson CL, Marsh WL. Inactivation of Kell blood group antigens by 2-aminoethylisothiouronium bromide. Br J Haematol 1982;51:107-15.
35. Edwards JM, Moulds JJ, Judd WJ. Chloroquine diphosphate dissociation of antigen-antibody complexes: a new technique for phenotyping red cells with a positive direct antiglobulin test. Transfusion 1982;22:59-61.
36. Masouredis SP, Sudora E, Mahan L, Victoria EJ. Quantitative immunoferritin microscopy of Fy^a, Fy^b, Jk^a, U, and Di^b antigen site numbers on human red cells. Blood 1980;56:969-77.
37. Williams D, Johnson CL, Marsh WL. Duffy antigen changes on red blood cells stored at low temperature. Transfusion 1981;21:357-9.
38. Dunstan RA, Simpson MB, Rosse WF. Erythrocyte antigens on human platelets. Absence of Rh, Duffy, Kell, Kidd and Lutheran antigens. Transfusion 1984;24:243-6.
39. Cedergren B, Giles CM. An Fy^xFy^x individual found in northern Sweden. Vox Sang 1973;24:264-6.
40. Habibi B, Perrier P, Salmon C. HD50 assay evaluation of the antigen Fy3 depression in Fy^x individuals. J Immunogenet 1980;7:191-3.
41. Oberdorfer CE, Kahn B, Moore V, Zelenski K, Øyen R, Marsh WL. A second example of anti-Fy3 in the Duffy blood group system. Transfusion 1974;14:608-11.
42. Buchanan DI, Sinclair M, Sanger R, Gavin J, Teesdale P. An Alberta Cree Indian with a rare Duffy antibody, anti-Fy3. Vox Sang 1976;30:114-21.
43. Kosinski KS, Molthan L, White L. Three examples of anti-Fy3 produced in Negroes. Rev Fr Transfus Immunohematol 1984;27:619-24.

44. Oakes J, Taylor D, Johnson C, Marsh WL. Fy3 antigenicity of blood of newborns (letter). Transfusion 1978;18:127.
45. DiNapoli J, Garcia A, Marsh WL, Dreizin D. A second example of anti-Fy5. Vox Sang 1976;30:308-11.
46. Chan-Shu SA. The second example of anti-Duffy[5]. Transfusion 1980;20:358-60.
47. Hutcheson JB, Haber JM, Kellner A. A hazard of repeated blood transfusions. Hemolytic reaction due to antibodies to the Duffy (Fy^a) factor. JAMA 1952;149:274-5.
48. Pineda AA, Brzica SM Jr, Taswell HF. Hemolytic transfusion reaction: Recent experience in a large blood bank. Mayo Clinic Proc 1978;53:378-90.
49. Freiesleben E. Fatal hemolytic transfusion reaction due to anti-Fy^a (Duffy). Acta Pathol Microbiol Scand 1951;29:283-6.
50. Badakere SS, Bhatia HM. A fatal transfusion reaction due to anti-Duffy (Fy^a). Indian J Med Sci 1970;24:562-4.
51. Boyland IP, Mufti GJ, Hamblin TJ. Delayed hemolytic transfusion reaction caused by anti-Fy^b in a splenectomized patient (letter). Transfusion 1982;22:402.
52. Badekere SS, Bhatia HM, Sharma RS, Bharucha Z. Anti-Fy^b (Duffy) as a cause of transfusion reaction. Indian J Med Sci 1970;24:565-7.
53. Ginsburg JC, Singer MA. Role of the Duffy A antigen in kidney transplantation (letter). N Engl J Med 1978;299(14):775.
54. Hunt ALC. Erythroblastosis fetalis due to anti-Fy^a in Salisbury, Rhodesia. Am J Med Tech 1967;33:479-81.
55. Greenwalt TJ, Sasaki T, Gajewski M. Further examples of hemolytic disease of the newborn due to anti-Duffy (anti-Fy^a). Vox Sang 1959;4:138-43.
56. Carreras-Vescio LA, Farina D, Rogido M, Sola A. Hemolytic disease of the newborn caused by anti-Fy^b (letter). Transfusion 1987;27:366.
57. Mourant AE, Kopec AC, Domaniewska-Sobczak K. The distribution of the human blood groups and other polmorphisms. London: Oxford Press, 1976.
58. Paul B. Duffy blood group distribution in Malawi. Trans R Soc Trop Med Hyg 1983;77(6):877.
59. Hitzeroth HW, Bender K, Burckhardt K. South African Negroes: serogenetic polymorphisms (ABO, Rhesus, MNS, Duffy and Kell) and inter-ethnic genetic distances. Acta Anthropogenet 1982;6(3):171-93.

60. Lewis M, Kaita H, Chown B. The Duffy blood group system in Caucasians. A further population sample. Vox Sang 1972;23:523-7.
61. Okubo Y, Yamaguchi H, Seno T, Yoshimura K, Tanaka M, Yokota T. Some rare blood group phenotypes in Japanese. Proceedings of the XV Congress. Paris: International Society for Blood Transfusion, 1978.
62. Chandanayingyong D, Sasaki TT, Greenwalt TJ. Blood groups of the Thais. Transfusion 1967;7:269-76.
63. Simmons RT, Graydon JJ. Population genetic studies in Australian Aborigines of the northern territory. Hum Biol Oceania 1971;1:23-53.
64. Sandler SG, Schiliro G, Russo A, Musumeci S, Rachmilewich EA. Blood group phenotypes and the origin of sickle cell hemoglobin in Sicilians. Acta Haematol 1978;60:350-7.
65. Sandler SG, Kravitz C, Sharon R, Hermoni D, Ezekiel E, Cohen T. The Duffy blood group system in Israeli Jews and Arabs. Vox Sang 1979;37:41-6.
66. Toivanen P, Hirvonen T. Antigens Duffy, Kell, Kidd, Lutheran and Xg^a on fetal red cells. Vox Sang 1973;24:372-6.
67. Palatnik M, Rowe AW. Duffy and Duffy-related human antigens in primates. J Hum Evol 1984;13:173-5.
68. Ruddle F, Riccuti F, McMorris FA, et al. Somatic cell genetic assignment of peptidase C and the *Rh* linkage group to chromosome A-1 in man. Science 1972;176:1429-31.
69. Paris Conference 1987. Human gene mapping 9 (in press).
70. Cook PJL, Page BM, Johnston AW, Stanford WK, Gavin J. Four further families informative for 1q and the Duffy blood group. Cytogenet Cell Genet 1978;22:378-80.
71. Guiloff RJ, Thomas PK, Contreras M, Armitage S, Schwarz G, Sedgwick EM. Linkage of autosomal dominant type 1 hereditary motor and sensory neuropathy to the Duffy locus on chromosome 1. J Neurol Neurosurg Psychiatry 1982;45:669-74.
72. Winter JH, Bennett B, Watt JL, et al. Confirmation of linkage between antithrombin III and Duffy blood group and assignment of AT3 to 1q22-q25. Ann Hum Genet 1982;46:29-34.
73. Race RR, Sanger R. Blood groups in man. 6th ed. Oxford: Blackwell Scientific, 1975.

74. Issitt PD, Issitt CH. Applied blood group serology. 2nd ed. Oxnard: Spectra Biologicals, 1975.
75. Salmon C, Cartron J-P, Rouger P. The human blood groups. New York: Masson Publishing, 1984.

In: Pierce, SR, and Macpherson, CR, eds.
Blood Group Systems: Duffy, Kidd and Lutheran
Arlington, VA: American Association
of Blood Banks, 1988

2

The Duffy Blood Group System: Biochemistry and Role in Malaria

Denise A. Valko, MS, MT(ASCP)SBB

INVESTIGATION OF DUFFY SYSTEM biochemistry began 10 years ago. Although the exact structure of the antigen(s) has not as yet been delineated, some important work has been done. It is by way of Duffy structures and those of other red cell membrane components, that the malarial protozoa attach to and invade red blood cells. An estimated million deaths per year result from malaria in Africa. If this system's biochemistry and its association with malarial invasion can be further defined, the burden that malaria has placed on mankind might be lessened. The recent advances in Duffy biochemistry and malarial invasion are the topic of this review.

Biochemistry

Table 2-1 lists several investigations of Duffy system biochemistry. Jensen and Furcht[1] were the first investigators to propose a location for Duffy system antigens. They solubilized red blood cell ghosts in sodium dodecyl sulfate (SDS) and subjected them to polyacrylamide gel electrophoresis (PAGE). The SDS-PAGE procedure separates individual membrane proteins according to molecular weight as they migrate through the gel. These investigators did not mention the Duffy phenotype of the red cells used, but concluded that "Duffy antigen" is located on or near glycophorin A, the MN sialoglycoprotein (SGP). Davies et al,[2] using soluble red blood cell extracts, reported Fy^a- and Fy^b-bearing structures to have an apparent molecular weight of 35 to 55 kD. The ability of the extract to inhibit anti-Fy^a and anti-Fy^b coincided with the Duffy phen-

---

Denise A. Valko, MS, MT(ASCP)SBB, Director, Technical Services, American Red Cross Blood Services, South Atlantic Region, Savannah, Georgia

Table 2-1. Summary of Duffy Biochemistry

Investigator	Year	Component	Molecular Weight (kD)	Characteristics
Jensen & Furcht[1]	1978	?		A: MN SGP
Davies et al[2]	1979	Fy^a Fy^b	35–55	S: heat at 56 C
Moore et al[3]	1982	Fy^a	39.5	A: MN SGP
			88	A: MN SGP, band 3
			64	?
Lisowska et al[6]	1983	Fy^a		Contains free thiol group
Hadley et al[7]	1984	Fy^a	35–43 (trailing edge to 66)	S: chymotrypsin, pronase, neuraminidase
Anstee[8]	1986	Fy^a	38.5	S: endo-B-galactosidase, endo F
Nichols et al[9]	1987	Fy6	46	S: chymotrypsin, papain, ficin

A = associated with; S = sensitive to

otypes of the red cells from which they were made. The isolated structures were heat sensitive in that they were denatured by heating at 56 C for 30 minutes and completely destroyed by heating at 65 C for 30 minutes.

Moore and coworkers[3] used radioiodinated, intact red blood cells (RBCs) incubated with human anti-Fy^a. The cells were solubilized and immune complexes isolated by adsorption to Staph protein A-sepharose. Staph protein A binds to the Fc portion of the antibody molecule. The complexes were eluted with SDS and subjected to PAGE. The presence of the ^{125}I-label was detected by autoradiography of the dried gels. They reported that Fy^a activity was associated with a substance of 39.5 kD. This structure had a mobility similar to PAS 2. (PAS 2 is one of the bands associated with the MN SGP.[4]) Fy^a activity was also associated with components with molecular weights of 64 and 88 kD, the latter of which had a mobility similar to PAS 1 and protein band 3.[3] (PAS 1 is also associated with the MN SGP[4,5]; band 3 is the major red cell membrane protein.) Other workers[6] have concluded that the Fy^a component contains a free thiol group. Reduced reactions were observed following treatment of intact red cells or isolated Fy(a+) membranes with sulfide-reducing agents.

Hadley et al[7] solubilized red cell membranes in SDS and subjected the extracts to PAGE and then immunoblotting. The blots were exposed to human anti-Fy^a, and antigen-antibody complexes were located using ^{125}I-labeled Staph protein A. The Fy^a antigen appeared as a broad band of apparent molecular weight of 35-43 kD with a diffuse trailing edge extending to 66 kD. Other indications that this was indeed the Fy^a antigen are that anti-Fy^a was affinity-purified from serum using the 35- to 43-kD region of the gel, and that material eluted from the band inhibited the agglutination of Fy(a+b−) red cells.

When the red cells used for study were treated with chymotrypsin and pronase (these enzymes destroy Fy^a activity on intact cells), the component was no longer present, indicating that it is protein in nature. In serological tests, trypsin does not destroy Fy^a antigenicity, so it came as no surprise when the band was still present following trypsin treatment of the ghosts. To determine whether the isolated component contained sialic acid, Fy(a+) red blood cell ghosts were treated with neuraminidase before SDS-PAGE, blotting and addition of anti-Fy^a. Neuraminidase treatment of the Fy^a ghosts did not remove Fy^a reactivity but altered its mobility. When boiled in a 5% solution of SDS containing 5% 2-mercaptoethanol, the 35- to 42-kD component aggregated, a property not observed with other proteins. The results with enzyme-treated cells, together with the explanation that the broadness of the band may be due to variable glycosylation, led these workers[7] to conclude that the Fy^a structure is glycoprotein in nature.

Anstee[8] treated intact Fy(a+) RBCs with endo-β-galactosidase, endo F and a mixture of the two. He found that the molecular weight of the leading edge of the Fy(a+) component was reduced from 38.5 to 33 kD following treatment with endo-β-galactosidase and to 26 kD following treatment with endo F. These enzymes cleave major sugar sequences attached to peptides. The results indicated that the Fy^a component may contain one or more N-glycosidically linked oligosaccharides which contribute between 40%-50% of the apparent molecular weight of the intact molecule. He also concluded that the Fy^a component is not associated with the red cell skeleton because the component is solubilized at low Triton X-100 concentrations.

Recently, Nichols et al,[9] using a murine monoclonal antibody, identified a component called Fy6 (see Chapter 1). The newly defined epitope has a distribution similar to that of the Fy3 antigen[10] [demonstrable on all red cells except for Fy(a−b−)]. It differs from Fy3 in that it is destroyed by chymotrypsin, ficin and papain. As discussed later, this structure may play a key role in malarial invasion. Using SDS-PAGE and Fy(a+b+), Fy(a+b−) and Fy(a−b+) RBCs, a rather broad band containing several sharper bands was observed. The strongest band seemed to be 46 kD. This band is not significantly different from that of the molecule Hadley et al[7] earlier showed to bear the Fy^a determinant. No band was seen using Fy(a−b−) cells.

Using Fy(a+) and/or Fy(b+) red cells, Nichols et al[9] estimated the number of Fy6 sites per red cell to be about 12,200. This value agrees closely with the earlier estimate[11] of approximately 13,300 Fy^a sites on Fy(a+b−) and 13,700 Fy^b sites on Fy(a−b+) red cells. Fy(a+b+) cells carry about 6900 Fy^a sites.

Thus, it appears that the structure containing Fy^a activity is not associated with the red cell skeleton, has a molecular weight of at least 35 kD with a trailing end extending to 66 kD and is probably on a structure not previously described. This component is sensitive to heat, certain proteases, neuraminidase, endo-β-galactosidase and endo F. It most probably is glycoprotein in nature.

Duffy and Malaria

Malaria and the *Plasmodium* Species Life Cycle

Malaria, which means bad air, was named because of the association of the disease with the odorous air of swamps, particularly at night. Human malaria is primarily caused by three species of *Plasmodium*: *vivax, falciparum* and *malariae*. A fourth species, *P. ovale*, is a rarer human parasite. *P. knowlesi*, which causes rapidly fatal infection in rhesus monkeys, causes relatively mild and temporary infection in man. Malaria has been, and is currently, a serious human disease. An estimated 150 million cases of malaria occur annually. The disease is found mainly in the tropics although it was formerly of considerable significance to the public health of the United States and Europe. *P. vivax* is the most common and the most widely distributed species. It has a 48-hour cycle of development in man. *P. falciparum* has a 40- to 48-hour cycle of development and causes a much more dangerous disease than the other species, but runs a shorter course. *P. malariae* is the cause of quartan malaria and it has a 72-hour cycle. Relapses are uncommon, but latent infection may persist for many years. *P. ovale* has been known only since 1922 and has a 48-hour cycle. There is no animal reservoir for any of these human parasites, except possibly chimpanzees for *P. malariae*. Malaria cannot, therefore, be acquired in uninhabited regions. For malaria to thrive there must be infected human beings, large numbers of man-biting female *Anopheles* sp. mosquitoes and easy contact between the two.

The complex life cycle of all species of *Plasmodium* is similar. (For a review, see Markell et al.[12]) The asexual life cycle is illustrated in Fig 2-1. Sporozoites are inoculated into man by the bites of a suitable species of female *Anopheles* mosquitoes. They do not enter the red blood cells immediately but leave the bloodstream and enter hepatic parenchymal cells. In *P. vivax* and *P. ovale* a proportion of the infecting sporozoites are believed to enter a resting stage before undergoing exoerythrocytic asexual multiplication. The resting stage of the parasite is known as a hypnozoite.

After a period of weeks or months, reactivation of the hypnozoite initiates asexual division. This type of reactivation is thought to bring about the relapses characteristic of *P. vivax* and *P. ovale*. Asexual multiplication in the liver results in the production of thousands of tiny merozoites in each infected cell. Rupture of these infected cells releases the merozoites

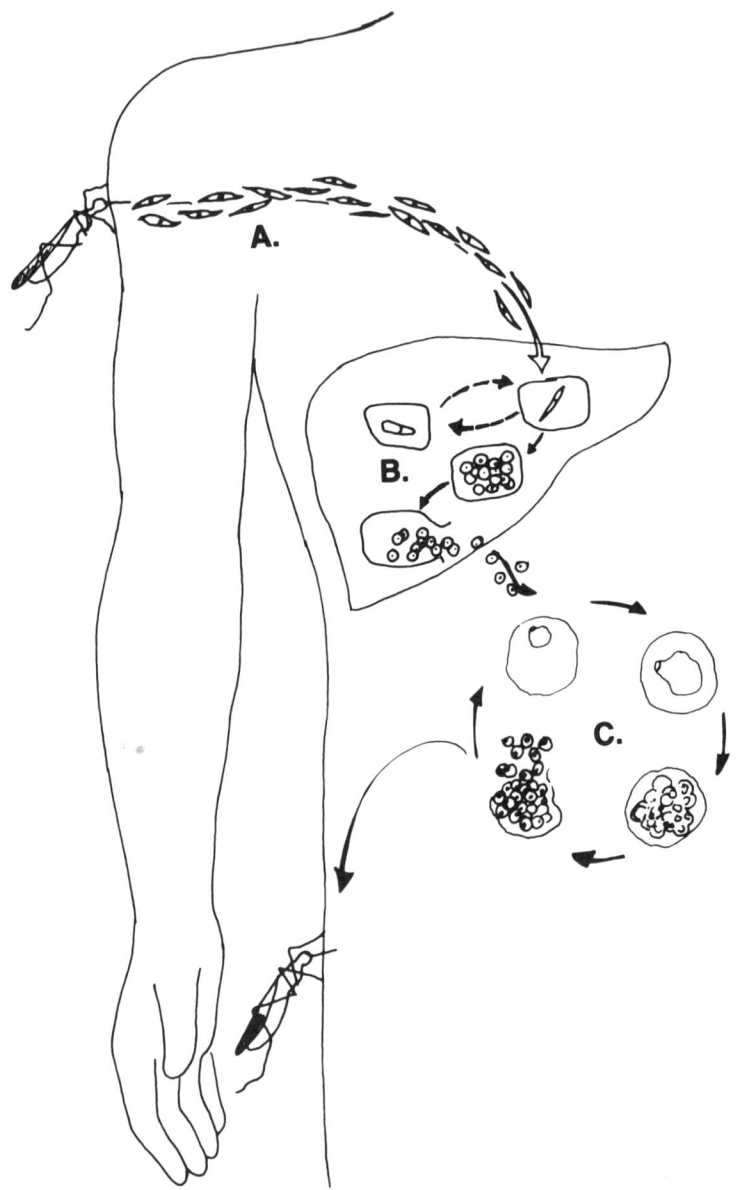

Figure 2-1. Asexual life cycle of the malarial parasite. (A) Sporozites injected by the biting mosquito are carried in the bloodstream to the liver. (B) Exoerythrocytic schizogony occurs in hepatic parenchymal cells. Merozoites are released which enter red blood cells or other liver cells. The dotted line represents the formation of a hypnozoite. (C) Red blood cell schizogony results in the formation of merozoites that will invade other RBCs or the eventual formation of gametocytes which are ingested by mosquitoes.

into the circulation to invade red blood cells or, as believed by some, other liver cells. In the red cells, the merozoites undergo growth and nuclear division. This tends to occur synchronously in a large number of red cells and, depending on the species, takes 48-72 hours. Inside a red cell, a merozoite develops into either an asexual parasite or a sexual gametocyte. Asexual parasites develop sequentially into ringforms, trophozoites and schizonts. These schizonts, when liberated, are called merozoites and enter a fresh red cell where the process is repeated.

After a few generations, some of these merozoites do not undergo nuclear division, but develop into a uninucleate organism called a gametocyte. When male and female gametocytes are taken up by a mosquito, they enter the gut where they develop into gametes and undergo fertilization. The resulting zygote undergoes numerous cell divisions and forms a bundle of spindle-shaped cells called sporozoites. These localize in the mosquito's salivary glands and are injected into the human bloodstream when the mosquito takes a blood meal. The cycle then repeats itself.

Clinical manifestations of the disease begin at the time of the bursting of the red cells. Malarial pigment, a degradation product of hemoglobin, and other waste products are released into the bloodstream and deposited in organs and under the skin. The characteristic paroxysms of chills and fever are felt at this time.

Since these protozoa are obligate intracellular parasites, the means of entry into red cells is crucial to their survival. Considerable work has been done in an attempt to identify the red cell surface structures and parasite components important for invasion.

Malarial Associations with Duffy Blood Group Antigens

Since 1955, it has been known that a high percentage of American and African Blacks were completely resistant to blood-induced infections with P. vivax.[13] In that same year, Sanger et al[14] reported that the majority of American and African Blacks were Fy(a−b−). Since the Fy(a−b−) phenotype is extremely rare in other racial groups without Black admixture,[15] the Duffy system antigens appeared to be the most likely candidates for malarial receptors.

In Vitro Studies Using P. knowlesi

Since P. vivax could not be cultured in vitro, the original work done by Miller et al[16-18] used P. knowlesi, a simian malarial parasite which invades human red blood cells. In brief, enzyme-treated and untreated human red cells were mixed with merozoite-infected rhesus red cells. The human red blood cells were from White and Black Fy(a+) and/or Fy(b+) individuals and from Black Fy(a−b−) individuals. The average invasion frequency for Fy(a+) and/or Fy(b+) nonenzyme-treated red cells was 80.3 parasitized cells per 1000. Only 2.2 parasitized cells per 1000 were observed in Fy(a−b−) cells.[16] The loss of susceptibility to invasion was directly correlated with the enzymatic removal of the Duffy blood group determinant by chymotrypsin and pronase.[18]

It was also shown that chymotrypsin did not just nonspecifically block invasion of the merozoite, but actually cleaved the Duffy protein.[19] Using inactivated chymotrypsin of the same strength, no reduction of invasion was observed. Trypsin- and neuraminidase-treated red cells, however, were invaded with the same frequency as untreated cells.[18] The lack of resistance shown by neuraminidase treatment indicated that the red cell negative surface charge was unrelated to susceptibility. Attempts to block invasion by adding red cell membrane components to the culture medium were unsuccessful.[18] Reduction in invasion was shown, however, by adding anti-Fy^a to Fy(a+) cells before adding the infective cells.[16] Red cells from three rare non-Black Fy(a−b−) persons were also resistant to invasion by *P. knowlesi*.[20] It would be of interest to test the red cells from these rare individuals for the presence of the Fy6 epitope.[9] Table 2-2 summarizes Duffy system antibody reactions using enzyme-treated and untreated human red blood cells. The susceptibility of these RBCs to invasion by *P. knowlesi* and *P. vivax* is also listed.

In Vivo Studies Using P. vivax

Miller et al[21] showed that Fy(a−b−) red cells were resistant to invasion by *P. vivax*. Since *P. vivax* could not (until recently[9]) be cultured in vitro, it was not possible to study invasion directly. They[21] determined the Duffy blood type of volunteers who had participated in malarial studies involving *P. vivax*. Five Fy(a−b−) Blacks were resistant to infection while the remaining six Blacks and five Whites who were Fy(a+) and/or Fy(b+) contracted malaria. Some of these same workers[22] determined the Duffy type of 13 Blacks who were infected with *P. vivax* while serving in Vietnam. All were Fy(a+) and/or Fy(b+). The chance that 13 of 13 would be positive for one of the Duffy antigens by chance alone is $p<0.001$.

A third in vivo study[23] involved testing 420 persons living in Honduras for Duffy type, antibodies to malarial parasites

Table 2-2. Reactions of Various Duffy System Antibodies with Enzyme-Treated and Untreated Human Red Blood Cells and Susceptibility to Malarial Invasion[9,16,18,20]

	Fy^a	Fy^b	Anti-Fy3	Fy5	Fy6*	P. knowlesi	P. vivax
Untreated	+	0	+	+	+	S	S
	0	+	+	+	+	S	S
	+	+	+	+	+	S	S
Black, untreated	0	0	0	0	0	R	R
Rare, non-Black, untreated	0	0	0	+	NT	R	NT
Rh$_{null}$ (amorph)	0	+	+	0	+	NT	NT
Rh$_{null}$ (regulator)	+	+	+	0	+	NT	NT
Fy(a+b+):C,P	0	0	+	+	0	R	NT
Fy(a+b+):T,N	+	+	+	+	+	S	NT
Fy(a−b−):T	0	0	0	0	NT	S	NT

S = successful invasion; R = resistance to invasion; C = chymotrypsin; P = pronase; T = trypsin; N = neuraminidase; NT = not tested; *murine monoclonal antibody

and infection with *P. vivax* or *P. falciparum*. Positive indirect fluorescent antibody (IFA) titers for *P. falciparum* were almost equally distributed between those with and those without Duffy system antigens. Positive IFA titers for *P. vivax*, however, were demonstrated almost exclusively in those with Duffy antigens. The authors offer very plausible reasons for the three positive IFA titers to *P. vivax* in Fy(a−b−) persons. The *P. falciparum* infections occurred equally in those with and those without Duffy system antigens. All active *P. vivax* infections, however, were from individuals positive for one of the Duffy antigens.

An Early Hypothesis, Discrepancies and Possible Resolutions

Miller et al[16] hypothesized that the Fy^a and Fy^b determinants were the receptors for invasion by *P. knowlesi* and *P. vivax*. Although this seemed like a logical conclusion at the time, there was some information that did not fit into this simple

model. Following each of the three points below is a possible explanation for the apparent discrepancy.
1. Although Fy(a−b−) red cells were not invaded by *P. knowlesi*, the merozoites do attach and cause widespread deformation of the cells.[24]
   Explanation: P. knowlesi merozoites attach to Fy(a−b−) as well as Fy(a+) and/or Fy(b+) red cells.[16, 17] The attachment site is presumed the same regardless of Duffy type. When the parasite attaches to Fy(a+) and/or Fy(b+) red cells, a junction, described below, occurs. The attachment with Fy(a−b−) cells, however, is instead characterized by fine fibrillar material connecting the parasite with the red cell.[25] The merozoite eventually detaches from the Fy(a−b−) RBCs and interacts with other red cells.[17] Apparently this attachment alone is sufficient to cause deformation.

   Two receptor sites appear to be involved. Site one is responsible for attachment and is present on red cells regardless of Duffy phenotype. Site two is the invasion site and is dependent on the presence of Fy^a and/or Fy^b (or Fy6?) antigens. Both sites are sensitive to chymotrypsin. Whether these sites are on the same or separate molecules is not known.[26] See Fig 2-2A for a hypothetical model of resistance following chymotrypsin treatment.
2. Trypsin- or neuraminidase-treated Fy(a−b−) red cells were invaded by *P. knowlesi*, although these cells lack demonstrable Fy^a or Fy^b sites.[20] In fact, Fy(a+) and/or Fy(b+) cells treated in the same manner were invaded at a higher rate.[20]
   Explanation: Some evidence suggests a third site[20, 26] or the blockage of the invasion site by a trypsin-sensitive masking molecule.[27] When Fy(a−b−) cells are treated with neuraminidase or trypsin, negatively charged sialic acid and sialoglycoprotein are removed, respectively. In the absence of these charges, the merozoite is hypothesized[20, 26, 27] to be able to interact (attach and invade) with Fy(a−b−) red cells. Whether this site is in any way associated with the Duffy system is unknown.[26] (See Fig 2-2B.)
3a. Some New World monkeys have red cells that were susceptible to invasion by *P. knowlesi* although no Fy^a or Fy^b antigens could be found on these cells.[20]
   b. Chymotrypsin-treatment of the red cells of some Old World Fy(b+) monkeys and chimpanzees did not prevent invasion by *P. knowlesi*.[20] As mentioned earlier, chymotrypsin treatment of human Fy(b+) cells did render them resistant to invasion.[16, 20]
   Explanation: Correlating information about nonhuman

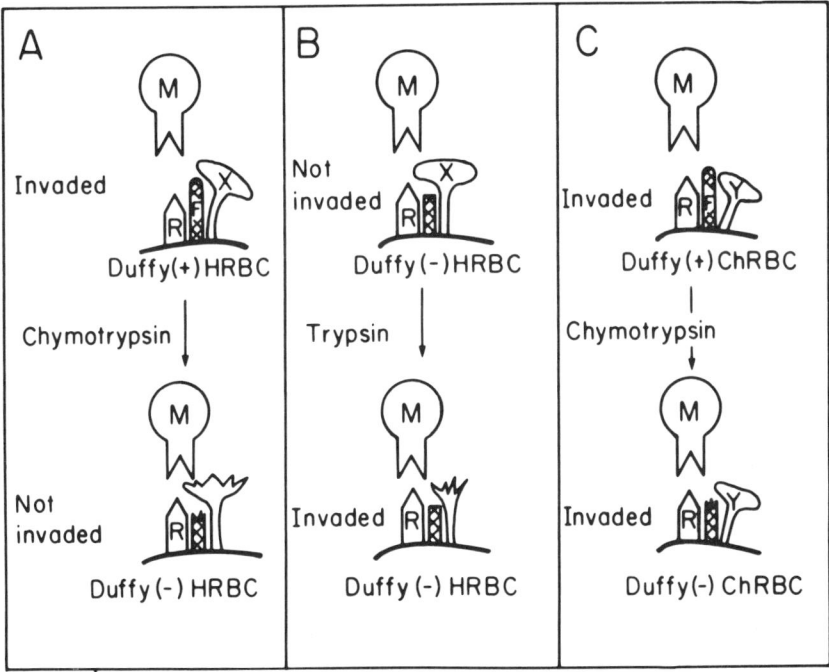

Figure 2-2. A hypothetical scheme for the interaction between P. knowlesi merozoites and Duffy-positive and -negative red blood cells. (A) A Duffy-positive human red blood cell which is invaded is converted by treatment with chymotrypsin to a Duffy-negative cell which is not invaded. (B) A Duffy-negative human red blood cell which is not invaded is converted by treatment with trypsin to a cell that remains Duffy-negative but is invaded. (C) A Duffy-positive chimpanzee red blood cell which is invaded is converted by treatment with chymotrypsin to a Duffy-negative cell which is still invaded. M, Merozoite; R, hypothetical junction receptor; F, Duffy determinants (Fy^a, Fy^b); X, hypothetical masking molecule on HRBC; HRBC, human red blood cell; ChRBC, chimpanzee red blood cell; Y, hypothetical masking molecule on ChRBC. Based on Miller et al[19] and Mason et al[20]. (Reproduced from *Int Rev Cytol*, 1985;96:212. Copyright permission, Academic Press.[27])

primates with that gathered studying human red cells is difficult and confusing.[9, 20, 26, 28, 29] Figure 2-2(A) and (C) show a possible explanation of how chymotrypsin-treated human and Old World monkey red cells could differ in invasion susceptibility. Some investigations have suggested that human and nonhuman red cells may demonstrate similar Duffy phenotypes using human-derived antisera, but not similar invasion patterns.[26, 29] This could be due to their being sufficiently similar for serological reactions but not for invasion. Another explanation could be that the human and nonhuman sites are different.

On the red cells of Old World monkeys (kra and rhesus are examples) and great apes (gorilla and chimpanzees are examples), Fy^b and Fy3 antigens are demonstrable. The red cells from these animals are susceptible to invasion by *P. knowlesi*. The red cells from the great apes react with anti-Fy6 and are invaded by *P. vivax*, whereas the red cells from the Old World monkeys are negative with anti-Fy6 and are not invaded by *P. vivax*.[9] The correlation between the presence of Fy6 and *P. vivax* seems to indicate that the receptors for *P. knowlesi* (Fy^b or Fy3?) and *P. vivax* (Fy6?) differ.

Perhaps to explain New World monkeys' susceptibility in the absence of Fy^a or Fy^b antigens, Fy3 is the receptor antigen. Hadley et al[26] were able to demonstrate the presence of Fy3 on New World monkey cells using adsorption and elution techniques. All three of the New World monkeys studied by Nichols et al[9] were positive for Fy3, but only two (*Saimiri sciureus* and *Aotus trivirgatus*) have been reported susceptible to invasion by *P. knowlesi*. The third species, *Cebus apella*, was not invaded by *P. knowlesi*. If Fy3 is the *P. knowlesi* invasion site for nonhuman primates, red cells from all monkeys should have been invaded. Some[26] have suggested that the *C. apella* red cells lack a different determinant necessary for invasion. These same two New World monkey species are invaded by *P. vivax* and have the newly defined Fy6 epitope. The third species (*C. apella*) lacks the Fy6 determinant and is accordingly not invaded by *P. vivax*. In summary, Fy3 appears to be the common denominator for invasion by *P. knowlesi* (except for *C. apella*) and Fy6 for *P. vivax*, with no exceptions.

Morphological Features of Invasion

Merozoite-Red Blood Cell Interactions

Using *P. knowlesi* and rhesus or human red blood cells and high-resolution light microscopy, Dvorak et al[24] recorded morphological changes of infected red cells. The initial attachment between the anterior end of the merozoite and the red cell results in a rapid and marked deformation of the red cell for 5-10 seconds. The actual invasion requires 10-20 seconds after which the red cell is again deformed. The second wave of deformation continues intermittently for 10-15 minutes. The merozoite then becomes very quiet and the red cell resumes its biconcave shape. Alternately, the infected red cell may crenate, swell and become a spherocyte. This process is accompanied by rapid spinning of the merozoite within the developing spherocyte. The spherocyte may lyse if swelling continues or return to its normal biconcave shape. In Fy(a−b−) red cells, the critical second stage of invasion does not occur and the merozoite eventually detaches and is capable of interacting with other red cells.[17]

Miller and colleagues,[25] using cytochalasin-B-treated malarial parasites, stopped invasion at the attachment phase in order to study the complicated events leading to invasion. The *P. knowlesi* merozoite released from the infected liver cells or red cells measures 2.0 × 1.5 μm. It is probably its outer membrane coat, consisting of short (20 nm) filaments projecting at right angles from the external membrane, which is responsible for initial adhesion to the red cell membrane.[30] The surface coat seems to be crucial to invasion since its absence is invariably associated with nonviability. Although this contact leads to overall deformation of the red cell, it does not result in localized invagination or invasion. Reorientation of the apical end and its apposition to the red cell membrane produces such an invagination.[30] The mechanism of apical orientation is unknown and could relate to receptor density, receptor distribution on the merozoite or contraction of the merozoite towards the apical region.[25] The point on the red cell membrane that is attached to the merozoite appears thickened and it is this thickened red cell membrane which forms a junction with the merozoite.[31] Figure 2-3 shows the thickened red cell membrane at the point of attachment.

The red cell and merozoite remain in contact only at the junction throughout the invasion process. This junction is defined morphologically by electron microscopy and consists of an electron dense area beneath the red cell membrane. The chemical basis of the junction is unknown. A pair of teardrop-shaped organelles called rhoptries and a few electron-dense micronemes are located in the apical region.[31] The rhoptries release their content into the red cell membrane causing the formation of vacuoles. The contents of these vacuoles are electron translucent although a few contain fine granular material.[30] Figure 2-3 shows some of these vacuoles.

The merozoite does not penetrate the red cell membrane but comes to lie within the parasitophorous vacuole. As the parasite proceeds, the junction subsequently forms a circumferential beltlike band around the merozoite which moves

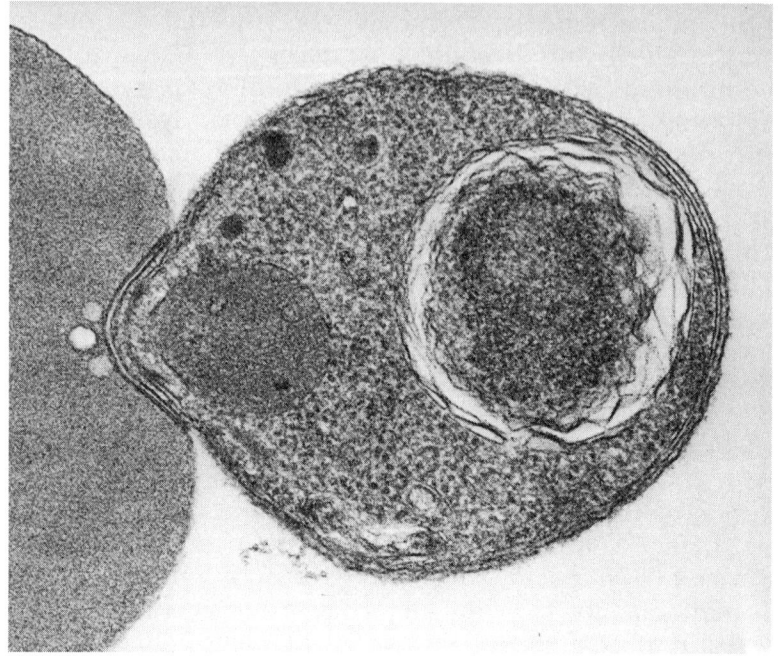

Figure 2-3. Electron micrograph showing the attachment between the apical end of a cytochalasin-B-treated merozoite and rhesus red cell. The red cell membrane is thickened at the attachment site. A few vacuoles are seen in the red cell cytoplasm and some of them are in contact with the invaginated red cell membrane. (× 50,000) (Reproduced from *J Exp Med*, 1979;149:178. Copyright permission, The Rockefeller University Press.[25])

from the apical to the caudal end of the parasite. This allows the parasite into the vacuole and subsequently the red cell.

The means by which the merozoite induces the red cell membrane to invaginate is not yet understood. Breuer[27] believes the binding of the merozoite to its appropriate receptor may result in disruption and inward collapse of the underlying membrane structure. This would allow the formation of the parasitophorous vacuole. Once the parasite is inside the red cell, the red cell undergoes a second wave of deformation and reseals.

The formation of a junction is absolutely essential to invasion. If attachment, but no invasion, occurs, electron micrographs show the red cell to be about 120-160 nm from the merozoite and connected by thin filaments measuring 3-5 nm.[25] Figure 2-4 is an electron micrograph of attachment between a merozoite and Fy(a−b−) human red blood cell.

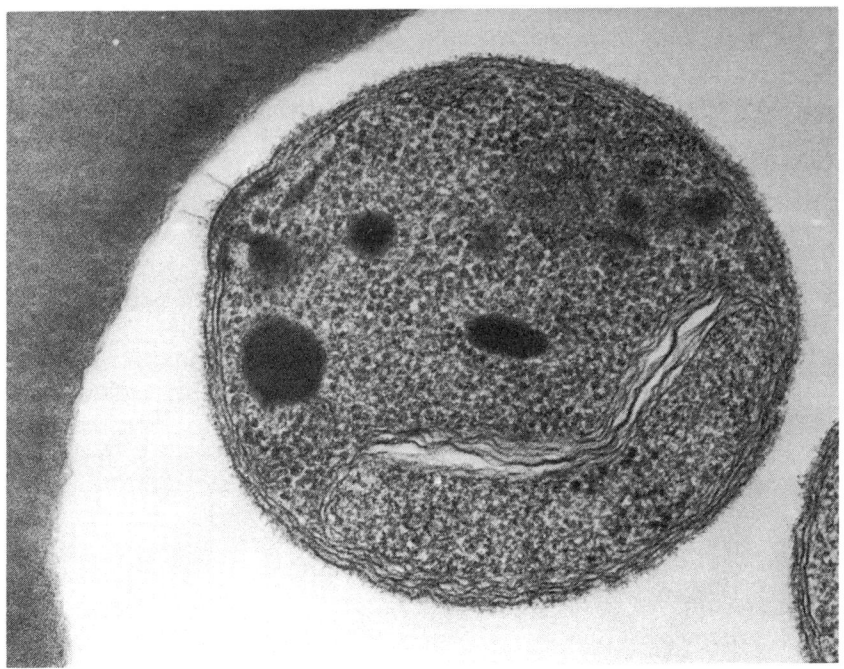

Figure 2-4. Electron micrograph showing that a cytochalasin-B-treated merozoite is connected with a Fy(a–b–) human red blood cell by two fine fibrils that are extending from the edge of the apical end. (Reproduced from *J Exp Med*, 1979;149:180. Copyright permission, Rockefeller University Press.[25])

Some have reported the presence of knobs[32] and new antigens[33] on the surface of red blood cells infected with mature *P. falciparum* merozoites. It is not known whether these components are derived directly from the parasite or from altered host components. Friedman et al[34] reported another interesting feature of *P. falciparum* invasion. They found that invasion was effectively inhibited by erythroglycan, a carbohydrate component of band 3. Involvement of this transmembrane protein might explain some of the radical alterations of the red cell cytoskeleton that accompany invasion.

Important Merozoite Proteins

Haynes and colleagues[35] and Haynes JD (personal communication) recently identified a parasite protein that appears to play a role in the red cell invasion process. Metabolically labeled *P. knowlesi* schizont-infected rhesus red blood cells were cultured. The culture supernatant was then incubated with uninfected human (or animal) test red cells, centrifuged and bound molecules eluted. The eluate was submitted to SDS-PAGE and analyzed by autoradiography. A 135-kD protein was found that bound to Fy(a+) and/or Fy(b+), but not to Fy(a−b−) red cells. This protein did not bind to human red cells that had been treated with chymotrypsin to remove Duffy antigens and render them resistant to invasion. They also found that the protein bound to the 35- to 43-kD region of blots prepared from Fy(a+) and Fy(b+), but not Fy(a−b−) red cell ghosts.

Although the protein consistently distinguished Fy^a and Fy^b on human red cells, in two instances red cells invaded by *P. knowlesi* did not bind the newly described protein. As discussed, trypsin-treated Fy(a−b−) red cells are invaded by *P. knowlesi*.[18] These cells, however, did not bind the 135-kD protein. Additionally, chymotrypsin-treated rhesus red cells were still invaded, although they do not have any demonstrable Fy^a or Fy^b antigens nor do they bind the 135-kD molecule. The enzymes may expose cryptic non-Duffy sites that allow invasion, by-passing the more usual (?) normal pathway requiring the 135-kD protein.

Haynes and coworkers (Haynes JD, personal communication) questioned the role of this protein. It could be responsible for one or more of the following: preparing red cells for invasion, activating merozoites by transmitting some sort of signal, acting as an adhesion molecule between the merozoite and red cell. It is probably not involved in the merozoite attachment seen with Fy(a−b−) red cells. These scientists also questioned why the protein was found in the culture supernatant and observed that it was only a small fraction of the total proteins present.

Camus and Hadley[36] identified a specific 175-kD protein in the supernatant of a *P. falciparum* culture which bound only to red cells susceptible to invasion by this parasite. Additionally, red cells treated with chymotrypsin at doses that do not inhibit merozoite invasion bound this protein. Trypsin- and neuraminidase-treated red cells are somewhat refractory to *P. falciparum* invasion (see below) and the identified component did not bind to these cells. These authors concluded that the binding of the 175-kD antigen to red cells correlates with their susceptibility to invasion and the protein may be a receptor that acts as a bridge between the red cell and the merozoite.

Some Questions Still Remain

Recent evidence[9] suggests that receptor sites for *P. knowlesi* and *P. vivax* may be distinct.

Fy3

The Fy3 antigen[10] is present on all Fy(a+) and/or Fy(b+) red cells and absent on Fy(a−b−) cells. With the exception of one type of New World monkey, Fy3 is the likely candidate for *P. knowlesi* invasion in nonhuman primates. Fy3 may not be the receptor in humans, however, since chymotrypsin treatment of Fy:3 cells blocks invasion of *P. knowlesi* but does not affect the Fy3 antigen.[20] If a masking molecule is present, as suggested by Breuer,[27] this would explain the resistance of these cells to invasion. Of course, the site on nonhuman primates and humans may not even be the same epitope as recognized by human antisera.

Fy5

The Fy5 antigen[37] resembles Fy3 but is absent from Rh_{null} red cells regardless of their Fy^a and Fy^b status. Fy5 is also present on the red cells of those rare Fy(a−b−) non-Black persons. Fy5 does not appear to be the human receptor for *P. knowlesi* since the Fy:5 red cells from these rare individuals are not invaded by *P. knowlesi*. These red cells must be tested for the Fy6 antigen and, if negative, submitted to in vitro *P. vivax* culture to rule out Fy5 as the *P. vivax* receptor.

Fy6

Limited evidence[9] indicates that the Fy6 antigen on both nonhuman primate and human red cells is the invasion site for *P. vivax*. Fy6 is not the invasion site for *P. knowlesi* on nonhuman primate cells, however, since the red cells from Old World monkeys are invaded by this parasite but are Fy:−6. The invasion site could be an epitope not yet identified but sterically influenced by specific Duffy system antigen presence or absence.

Malarial Associations with Other Red Cell Membrane Structures

P. falciparum and a Sialic-Acid-Dependent Site

In contrast to *P. vivax*, *P. falciparum* infects Black and White persons equally, regardless of Duffy type, suggesting that the receptor for invasion may be different from that used by *P. vivax*. N-acetyl neuraminic acid (NeuNAc) or sialic acid is important for invasion by this malaria parasite, which involves glycophorins A and B, the sialoglycoproteins (SGPs) responsible for MN and SsU specificities, respectively. (See Issitt[29, 38] and Anstee[39] for reviews of these structures.)

MN and Ss SGPs

The MN SGP is sensitive to many proteases and contains about 60% of the red-cell-bound neuraminidase-sensitive sialic acid. Cells lacking the MN SGP are called En(a−). Several workers[26, 40-42] tested normal RBCs and those that lacked certain blood group determinants and found that all cells, including Fy(a−b−) cells, were invaded normally by *P. falciparum* except for En(a−) red cells which showed a reduced invasion. The amount of resistance varied dependent on the parasite strain used. Pasvol et al[41] also demonstrated that En(a+) cells that had been sensitized with anti-En^a had reduced invasion. Reduced invasion of normal red cells also resulted following treatment with trypsin[26, 40] and neuraminidase,[40] whereas chymotrypsin did not cause a reduction.[40] Invasion was also reduced following the addition of soluble glycophorin A or Fab' fragments against glycophorin A.[43] Since infection of En(a−) cells was not completely inhibited, the MN SGP cannot be the sole receptor for invasion.

Pasvol et al[44] observed reduced invasion when studying the red cells of the MN-Ss SGP hybrid, AG. The red cells of individuals genetically M^gM^g (lacking side chains at amino acids 2,3 and 4) and MM^c (M^c is the intermediate antigen between the M and N SGPs) demonstrated normal invasion.[45]

Some workers[42, 44] found reduced invasion of S−s−U− cells when compared with normal cells, whereas others[46] did not observe a reduction. This discrepancy may be due to heterogeneity of either red cells or parasites.[26] When these workers[42, 46] treated S−s−U− cells with trypsin, as much as 90% reduction of invasion was observed. These findings suggest that sites for invasion are found on the MN SGP, Ss SGP and at least one other (trypsin-resistant) component.

Glycophorin-C-deficient red cells demonstrate reduced malarial invasion.[47] This is consistent with the involvement of sialic acid as an important receptor for invasion.

Tn and Cad Red Blood Cells

Tn-activated and Cad red blood cells have altered SGP-borne tetrasaccharides and consequently have been shown to have increased resistance to *P. falciparum* invasion. Tn red cells lack galactose and sialic acid on the O-linked tetrasaccharides of the MN and Ss SGPs. Although much of the N-acetyl neuraminic acid is removed, Tn cells have 49-68% of the amount of sialic acid normally found on red cells.[48] Many workers have shown that Tn cells are resistant to *P. falciparum* invasion, although the degree of reduction in invasion may depend on the strain of parasite used.[45, 49] This evidence, together with the knowledge that neuraminidase treatment reduces invasion, is further support that sialic acid contributes in some way to *P. falciparum* invasion.

Cad-positive red cells have a normal amount of sialic acid, but have an extra carbohydrate residue (N-acetylgalactosamine) attached to each chain branching from the MN and Ss SGPs. Cad cells also demonstrate reduced invasion.[45] It has been suggested that the extra sugar molecule changes the orientation of the sialic acid so that it is not recognized by the parasite.[45]

M^kM^k Red Blood Cells

M^kM^k red cells lack both the MN and Ss SGPs and have been studied by Hadley et al[26, 50] using two strains of *P. falciparum* (Camp and 7G8). Invasion rates obtained with nonenzyme-treated M^kM^k cells using these strains were 20% and greater than 50%, respectively, of the rates obtained with normal red cells. Invasion of M^kM^k RBCs by the sialic-acid-dependent Camp parasite was markedly reduced by neuraminidase treatment but unaffected by trypsin. In contrast, neuraminidase treatment had little effect on invasion by the 7G8 parasite, but trypsin treatment of these cells reduced invasion greatly.

The Wr(a+b−) Phenotype

Although initial tests[44] indicated reduced invasion of Wr(a+b−) red cells by *P. falciparum*, many subsequent studies[51-55] found them fully susceptible to invasion. Perhaps the cells used in the initial investigation had been damaged during transport or storage and were suboptimal. Although reduced invasion of Wr(b+) RBCs was also observed following the addition of immune and monoclonal antibodies with anti-Wr^b specificity,[44] other workers[51] found this not to be so. The Wr^b antigen, therefore, is no longer considered an important component for *P. falciparum* invasion.

As can be seen, evaluating invasion rates by *P. falciparum* with different types of red cells is more complicated than that of *P. vivax*. Evidence suggests that:

1. The MN and Ss SGPs, with their accompanying sialic acids, appear not to be required for invasion by *P. falciparum*, although more efficient invasion occurs if these structures are present.
2. The degree of dependence on NeuNAc for invasion differs among various strains.
3. The Camp strain uses a trypsin-insensitive site (Ss SGP?), which apparently is not used by the 7G8 strain. (This would explain normal invasion by the former strain following trypsin treatment.)

All of the above information leads to an additional conclusion that there exist sialic-acid-dependent and -independent sites and trypsin-sensitive and -resistant sites and combinations of the above.

P. Falciparum and a Sialic-Acid-Independent Site

Since some invasion does occur using red cells devoid of sialic acid, there must be a sialic-acid-independent invasion site. After reviewing his work and that of others, Hadley et al[26] concluded that a sialic-acid-independent, neuraminidase-resistant, trypsin-sensitive site located on a molecule other than the MN or Ss SGPs or on a site common to both the MN SGP and another trypsin-sensitive component exists. *P. falciparum* probably presents two receptors: one binds to a sialic-acid-dependent ligand, and one binds to a sialic-acid-independent ligand. Since there is such a difference in invasion rates among different lines of *P. falciparum*, the quantity or affinity of the receptors for the sialic-acid-independent site may differ. Whether or not this site is on glycophorin C, as suggested by some,[26, 42] requires further investigation.

Development of a Malarial Vaccine

Recently accumulated knowledge may soon help in the better management and eradication of malaria. Each stage in the *Plasmodium* life cycle is antigenically and morphologically distinct and could be interrupted by a vaccine. A sporozoite vaccine should prevent development of hepatic schizonts and the subsequent blood invasion. A vaccine against one of the many merozoite proteins should stop or limit the multiplication of malaria parasites in the blood. This would prevent or reduce clinical symptoms and may slow transmission. The third type of vaccine should prevent fertilization of female gametes by male gametes or interfere with the growth of the fertilized zygote. Along with the gametes, the mosquito would ingest some of the host blood containing specific antibodies to the gametes or oocyst. This last type of vaccine would not necessarily help the host, but would block the transmission of malaria in a community.

Great strides have been made in human malarial vaccine production.[56-58] After administering a recombinant DNA *P. falciparum* sporozoite vaccine to 15 human volunteers, Ballou et al[59] concluded that improvements needed to be made before further field trials took place. It has also been shown that a vaccine must be able to elicit responses superior to that of naturally occurring antibodies.[60]

Conclusion

Now that progress is being made in Duffy-antigen biochemistry and elucidation of red blood cell invasion receptors and merozoite attachment sites, it is hoped that this information will continue to help in determining the best route to pursue in the production of a successful vaccine.

Acknowledgments

I am indebted to my secretary, Kristie Schandolph, who read my hieroglyphic handwriting and was very patient with me through all of my many revisions. I thank Mary McGinniss and Drs. Hadley and Miller for their suggestions. I also thank Dr. Haynes for sharing some of his unpublished work. I am grateful to Dr. Aikawa for providing photographs of his merozoite-red-blood- cell electron micrographs. Last, I owe special gratitude to my friend and colleague Mary Ann Spivey who scrutinized the manuscript.

References

1. Jensen NH, Furcht LT. Localization of the Duffy antigen on the red cell membrane components (abstract). Transfusion 1978;18:643.
2. Davies DM, Hall SJ, Graham HA, Chachowski R. The isolation and partial characterization of Duffy antigens from human red cells (abstract). Transfusion 1979;19:638.
3. Moore S, Woodrow CF, McClelland DBL. Isolation of membrane components associated with human red cell

antigens Rh (D), (c), (E) and Fy^a. Nature 1982;295:529-31.
4. Marton LSG, Garvin JE. Subunit structure of the major human erythrocyte glycoprotein: depolymerization by heating ghosts with sodium dodecylsulfate. Biochem Biophys Res Commun 1973;52:1457-62.
5. Fairbanks G, Steck TL, Wallach DFH. Electrophoretic analysis of the major polypeptides of the human erythrocyte membrane. Biochemistry 1971;10:2606-17.
6. Lisowska E, Duk M, Wasniowska K. Duffy antigens: observations on biochemical properties. In: Carton J-P, Rouger P, Salmon Ch, eds. Red cell membrane glycoconjugates and related genetic markers. Paris: Librairie Arnette, 1983:87-96.
7. Hadley TJ, David PH, McGinniss MH, Miller LH. Identification of an erythrocyte component carrying the Duffy blood group Fy^a antigen. Science 1984;223:597-9.
8. Anstee DJ. Blood group active components of the human cell membrane. In: Garratty G, ed. Red cell antigens and antibodies. Arlington, VA: American Association of Blood Banks, 1986:1-15.
9. Nichols ME, Rubinstein P, Barnwell J, de Cordoba SR, Rosenfield RE. A new human Duffy blood group specificity defined by a murine monoclonal antibody. Immunogenetics and association with susceptibility to *Plasmodium vivax*. J Exp Med 1987;166:776-85.
10. Albrey JA, Vincent EER, Hutchinson J, et al. A new antibody, anti-Fy3, in the Duffy blood group system. Vox Sang 1971;20:29-35.
11. Masouredis SP, Sudora E, Mahan L, Victoria EJ. Quantitative immunoferritin microscopy of Fy^a, Fy^b, Jk^a, U and Di^b antigen site numbers on human red cells. Blood 1980;56:969-77.
12. Markell EK, Voge M, John DT. Medical parasitology. 6th ed. Philadelphia: WB Saunders, 1986.
13. Young MD, Eyles DE, Burgess RW, Jeffrey GM. Experimental testing of the immunity of Negroes to *Plasmodium vivax*. J Parasitol 1955;41:315-8.
14. Sanger R, Race RR, Jack J. The Duffy blood groups of New York Negroes: the phenotype Fy(a−b−). Br J Haematol 1955;1:370-4.
15. Mourant AE, Kopec AC, Domaniewska-Sobczak K. The distribution of the human blood groups and other polymorphisms. 2nd ed. London: Oxford University Press, 1976.

16. Miller LH, Mason SJ, Dvorak JA, McGinniss MH, Rothman IK. Erythrocyte receptors for (*Plasmodium knowlesi*) malaria: Duffy blood group determinants. Science 1975;189:561-63.
17. McGinniss MH, Miller LH. Malaria erythrocyte receptors and the Duffy blood group system. In: Steane EA, ed. Cellular antigens and disease. Washington, DC: American Association of Blood Banks, 1977:67-77.
18. Miller LH, Dvorak JA, Shiroishi T, Durocher JR. Influence of erythrocyte membrane components on malaria merozoite invasion. J Exp Med 1973;138:1597-601.
19. Miller LH, Shiroishi T, Dvorak JA, Durocher JR, Schrier BK. Enzymatic modification of the erythrocyte membrane surface and its effect on malarial merozoite invasion. J Mol Med 1975;1:55-63.
20. Mason SJ, Miller LH, Shiroishi T, Dvorak JA, McGinniss MH. The Duffy blood group determinants: their role in the susceptibility of human and animal erythrocytes to *Plasmodium knowlesi* malaria. Br J Haematol 1977;36:327-35.
21. Miller LH, Mason SJ, Clyde DF, McGinniss MH. The resistance factor to *Plasmodium vivax* in Blacks. The Duffy blood group genotype, *FyFy*. N Engl J Med 1976;295:302-4.
22. Miller LH, McGinniss MH, Holland PV, Sigmon P. The Duffy blood group phenotype in American Blacks infected with *Plasmodium vivax* in Vietnam. Am J Trop Med Hyg 1978;27:1069-72.
23. Spencer HC, Miller LH, Collins WE, et al. The Duffy blood group and resistance to *Plasmodium vivax* in Honduras. Am J Trop Med Hyg 1978;27:664-70.
24. Dvorak JA, Miller LH, Whitehouse WC, Shiroishi T. Invasion of erythrocytes by malaria merozoites. Science 1975;187:748-50.
25. Miller LH, Aikawa M, Johnson JG, Shiroishi T. Interaction between cytochalasin B-treated malarial parasites and erythrocytes: Attachment and junction formation. J Exp Med 1979;149:172-84.
26. Hadley TJ, McGinniss MH, Klotz FW, Miller LH. Blood group antigens and invasion of erythrocytes by malaria parasites. In: Garratty G, ed. Red cell antigens and antibodies. Arlington, VA: American Association of Blood Banks, 1986:17-33.
27. Breuer WV. How the malaria parasite invades its host cell, the erythrocyte. Int Rev Cytol 1985;96:191-238.

28. Marsh WL. Present status of the Duffy blood group system. CRC Crit Rev Clin Lab Sci 1975;5:387-412.
29. Issitt PD. Applied blood group serology. 3rd ed. Miami: Montgomery Scientific, 1985.
30. Bannister LH, Butcher GA, Dennis ED, Mitchell GH. Structure and invasive behavior of *Plasmodium knowlesi* merozoites in vitro. Parasitology 1975;71:483-91.
31. Aikawa M, Miller LH, Johnson JG, Rabbege J. Erythrocyte entry by malarial parasites. A moving junction between erythrocyte and parasite. J Cell Biol 1978;77:72-82.
32. Sherman, IW. Membrane structure and function of malaria parasites and the infected erythrocyte. Parasitology 1985;91:689-95.
33. Marsh K, Howard RJ. Antigens induced on erythrocytes by *P. falciparum*: expression of diverse and conserved determinants. Science 1986;231:150-3.
34. Friedman MJ, Fukuda M, Laine RA. Evidence for a malarial parasite interaction site on the major transmembrane protein of the human erythrocyte. Science 1985;228:75-7.
35. Haynes JD, Klotz FW, Miller LH. A 135- kilodalton receptor molecule from malaria parasites binds to a human erythrocyte ligand associated with Duffy antigens and correlates with invasion (abstract). Clin Res 1987;35:615A.
36. Camus D, Hadley TJ. A *Plasmodium falciparum* antigen that binds to host erythrocytes and merozoites. Science 1985;230:553-6.
37. Colledge KI, Pezzulich M, Marsh WL. Anti-Fy5, an antibody disclosing a probable association between the Rhesus and Duffy blood group genes. Vox Sang 1973;24:193-9.
38. Issitt PD. The MN blood group system. Cincinnati: Montgomery Scientific, 1981.
39. Anstee DJ. The blood group MNSs-active sialoglycoproteins. Semin Hematol 1981;18:13-31.
40. Miller LH, Haynes JD, McAuliffe FM, Shiroishi T, Durocher JR, McGinniss MH. Evidence for differences in erythrocyte surface receptors for the malarial parasites, *Plasmodium falciparum* and *Plasmodium knowlesi*. J Exp Med 1977;146:277-81.
41. Pasvol G, Wainscoat JS, Weatherall DJ. Erythrocytes deficient in glycophorin resist invasion by the malarial parasite *Plasmodium falciparum*. Nature 1982;297:64-6.

42. Facer CA. Erythrocyte sialoglycoproteins and *Plasmodium falciparum* invasion. Trans R Soc Trop Med Hyg 1983;77:524-30.
43. Perkins M. Inhibitory effects of erythrocyte membrane proteins on the in vitro invasion of the human malarial parasite (*Plasmodium falciparum*) into its host cell. J Cell Biol 1981;90:563-7.
44. Pasvol G, Jungery M, Weatherall DJ, Parsons SF, Anstee DJ, Tanner MJA. Glycophorin as a possible receptor for *Plasmodium falciparum*. Lancet 1982;2:947-50.
45. Cartron JP, Prou O, Luilier M, Soulier JP. Susceptibility to invasion of some human erythrocytes carrying rare blood group antigens. Br J Haematol 1983;55:639-47.
46. Howard RJ, Haynes JD, McGinniss MH, Miller LH. Studies on the role of red blood cell glycoproteins as receptors for invasion by *Plasmodium falciparum* merozoites. Mol Biochem Parasitol 1982;6:303-15.
47. Pasvol G, Anstee D, Tanner MJA. Glycophorin C and the invasion of red cells by *Plasmodium falciparum*. Lancet 1984;1:907-8.
48. Dahr W, Uhlenbruck G, Gunson HH, van der Hart M. Molecular basis of Tn-polyagglutinability. Vox Sang 1975;29:36-50.
49. Mitchell GH, Hadley TJ, McGinniss MH, Klotz FW, Miller LH. Invasion of erythrocytes by *Plasmodium falciparum* malaria parasites: evidence for receptor heterogeneity and two receptors. Blood 1986;67:1519-21.
50. Hadley TJ, Klotz FW, Pasvol G, et al. Falciparum malaria parasites invade erythrocytes that lack glycophorin A and B (M^kM^k). Strain differences indicate receptor heterogeneity and two pathways for invasion. J Clin Invest 1987;80:1190-3.
51. Hermentin P, David PH, Miller LH, Perkins ME, Pasvol G, Dahr W. Wright (a+b−) human erythrocytes and *Plasmodium falciparum* malaria. Blut 1985;50:75-80.
52. Facer CA, Mitchell GH. Wr^b negative erythrocytes are susceptible to invasion by malaria parasites (letter). Lancet 1984;2:758-9.
53. Schulman S, Vanderberg JP. Wright's b determinant, monoclonal antibodies, and *Plasmodium falciparum* merozoite invasion (letter). Lancet 1984;2:934-5.
54. Hermentin P, Enders B, Neunziger G, et al. Wr(a+b−) red blood cells are fully susceptible to invasion by *Plasmodium falciparum* (letter). Lancet 1984;2:466.

55. Cartron JP, Tounkara A, Prou O, Luilier M, Soulier JP. Wr^b antigen not required for invasion of human erythrocytes by *Plasmodium falciparum* (letter). Lancet 1984;2:466-7.
56. Miller LH, Howard RJ, Carter R, Good MF, Nussenzweig V, Nussenzweig RS. Research toward malaria vaccines. Science 1986;234:1349-56.
57. Bruce-Chwatt LJ. The challenge of malaria vaccine: trials and tribulations. Lancet 1987;1:371-3.
58. Walsh J. Human trials begin for malaria vaccine. Science 1987;235:1319-20.
59. Ballou WR, Hoffman SL, Sherwood JA, et al. Safety and efficacy of a recombinant DNA *Plasmodium falciparum* sporozoite vaccine. Lancet 1987;1:1277-81.
60. Hoffman SL, Oster CN, Plowe CV, et al. Naturally acquired antibodies to sporozoites do not prevent malaria: vaccine development implications. Science 1987;237:639-42.

In: Pierce, SR, and Macpherson, CR, eds.
Blood Group Systems: Duffy, Kidd and Lutheran
Arlington, VA: American Association
of Blood Banks, 1988

3

The Kidd Blood Group System: Serology and Genetics

Ruth Mougey, MT(ASCP)SBB

THE DISCOVERY OF THE Kidd blood group system came in that period of rapid advancement in blood group serology and transfusion therapy that followed the development of the antiglobulin test in 1945. This well-defined system has changed little from the 1950's when all major discoveries were made. Allen et al[1] described Jk^a in 1951, Plaut and colleagues[2] found the allele Jk^b in 1953 and Pinkerton et al[3] found the first example of a $Jk(a-b-)$ person in 1959. Since then, most reports on the Kidd system have concerned the propensity of these antibodies to cause either immediate or delayed hemolytic transfusion reactions and then to disappear without a trace.

To date no low frequency antigens have been associated with the Kidd system, and no person of a common Kidd phenotype has been found to have an alloantibody compatible only with $Jk(a-b-)$ red cells. This is a dramatic departure from most other blood group systems which have become amazingly complex in the last 15 years. Perhaps monoclonal antibodies will rescue this system from its dull niche, although interestingly enough, a monoclonal Kidd antibody has not been reported, further evidence of Kidd's resistance to change. In spite of this, the Kidd system is very important on a practical level and blood bankers need to be knowledgeable about its properties and requirements.

Genetics

Population studies and family studies with anti-Jk^a and anti-Jk^b showed that the genes are inherited in a straightforward Mendelian manner with the strength of the antigen depen-

---

Ruth Mougey, MT(ASCP)SBB, Director, Reference Laboratory, American Red Cross Blood Services, Badger Region, Madison, Wisconsin

Table 3-1. Phenotype and Frequencies

Tests with				Adult Phenotype Frequencies (%)		
Anti-Jk^a	Anti-Jk^b	Anti-Jk3	Phenotype	White[4]	Black[4]	Oriental[5,6]
+	0	+	Jk(a+b−)	26.3	51.1	23.22
+	+	+	Jk(a+b+)	50.3	40.8	49.94
0	+	+	Jk(a−b+)	23.4	8.1	26.84
0	0	0	Jk(a−b−)	<0.01	<0.01	0.9 to <0.1

dent on the presence of the gene in a single or double dose. The locus has three alleles: Jk^a, Jk^b and Jk. Whenever the Jk^a or Jk^b antigen is produced, the Jk3 antigen is also expressed (Table 3-1).[4-6] The Jk3 antigen is recognized by the antibody made by Jk(a−b−) persons. Anti-Jk3 should not be thought of as inseparable anti-Jk^a + anti-Jk^b; anti-Jk3 can be made by Jk$_{null}$ persons who have been sensitized only to the Jk^a or Jk^b antigen, yet their antibody reacts with a shared determinant present on cells of both phenotypes. No person has been found who has the Jk^a or Jk^b antigen but lacks the Jk3 antigen. However, two families have been found who have a Jk(a−b−)Jk:3 phenotype[7] (see below).

Humphrey and Morel[8] uncovered additional evidence about the expression of Jk3 when they studied the Kidd antigens of families with Jk(a−b−) members. They found that the dosage effect of the silent gene made persons of Jk^aJk or Jk^bJk genotypes have titration scores with anti-Jk^a or -Jk^b, similar to the heterozygous Jk^aJk^b control. When anti-Jk3 was used, however, the strength of the Jk3 antigen was like that of the homozygous $JkJk$ controls. They concluded that the Jk3 antigen was unaffected when the Jk gene was present in a single dose. This effect is not consistently noted in all reports[9] of Jk heterozygotes and may be related to differences in titration methods or to further heterogeneity of the Kidd blood group system genes.

In cases of disputed paternity, the Kidd system is fairly useful if both anti-Jk^a and -Jk^b are used; the exclusion rate is 0.19 in Whites and 0.16 in Blacks.[4] Unfortunately, pure, potent samples of the antibodies, especially anti-Jk^b, are rare, making paternity testing somewhat unreliable in the hands of a novice. Problems with weak reactions of some anti-Jk^b sera prompted studies by Boyd (unpublished observations

THE KIDD BLOOD GROUP SYSTEM 55

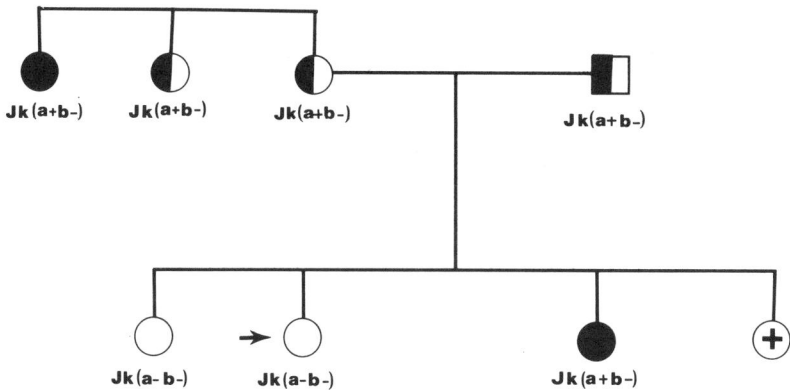

Figure 3-1. Part of the Rob family.[12] Strength of antigen determined by titration studies. ◐ = heterozygote, ○ = homozygote for *Jk*

cited in Issitt[10 (p 308)]), who tested a large number of samples with several different anti-Jk^b sera and found a great variation of antigen strengths but no evidence of a qualitative difference among weak Jk(b+) samples.

Whether the genes controlling the production of the Kidd antigens code for a protein which is the antigen, or act on a precursor is not known. However, with the rapid progress being made in biochemistry and molecular genetics, these questions may be answered in the near future.

The *Jk* allele to *Jk^a* and *Jk^b* does appear to be a truly amorphic gene in the family studies involving persons of the Jk(a−b−) phenotype.[9, 11, 12] In those studies, all parents of Jk$_{null}$ persons tested were either Jk(a+b−) or Jk(a−b+), and all offspring of Jk$_{null}$ persons were either Jk(a+b−) or Jk(a−b+) (Fig 3-1). In all but two instances, the Jk(a−b−) phenotype has been found in Far Eastern populations, with Polynesians having the highest frequency (0.9%).[6] At first the Jk(a−b−) phenotype was noted because the persons had formed anti-Jk3. However, a very useful observation was made by Heaton and McLoughlin,[13] who noticed that the red cells of a Jk(a−b−) patient did not lyse in 2M urea, but shrank and were counted as platelets by an automated instrument. The 2M-urea screening test easily detects Jk(a−b−) cells and, in the appropriate population, the procedure has found many new donors. Much of the progress made in the area of Kidd biochemistry concerns this phenomenon and will be covered in Chapter 4.

Habibi et al[12] reported the first Caucasian family with a Jk(a−b−) member in 1976 and Klarkowski (cited in

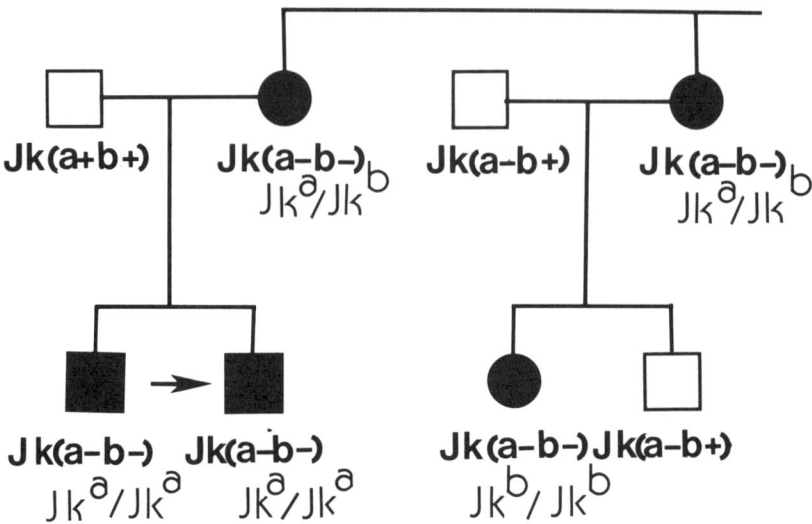

Figure 3-2. Part of the YS family.[7] Jk phenotype determined by absorbtion and elution studies. ● = presence of *In (Jk)*

Issitt[10 (p 653)]) found the second in 1983. The *Jk* gene is very rare in Caucasians but its presence had been suspected because of discrepant results of Kidd antigens in other family studies.[14] The inheritance of the *Jk* gene in Caucasians seems identical to that in other Jk$_{null}$ families.

A suppressor gene that affects Jk antigen expression has also been hinted at in some families,[15] but the data were in no way as convincing as the dramatic discovery by Okubo et al[7] of a dominant suppressor of Kidd antigens. In two unusual Japanese families they found by 2M-urea screening what appeared to be Jk(a−b−) individuals but who were later shown to react weakly with anti-Jk3 and to absorb and elute anti-Jk^a or -Jk^b. The inheritance of the suppressor appears to be dominant. None of the six persons with this new type of Jk$_{null}$ has made anti-Jk3 (Fig 3-2).

This apparently dominant suppression of Kidd antigens is similar to the *In(Lu)* suppression of the Lutheran system and the suppressor gene has been called *In(Jk)*. Like the amorphic Jk(a−b−) red cells, the *In(Jk)* red cells do not readily lyse in 2M urea, although they are not quite as resistant to hemolysis as the amorphic type. Although the resemblance between the Kidd suppression and the *In(Lu)* (or *Syn1*) suppression is very interesting, there are not enough data to speculate on the precise nature of this type of suppression.

Chromosome Assignment

The *Kidd* locus is a very mobile one if the literature is to be believed. In 1973, Shokeir et al[16] reported that the *Kidd* locus might be on the distal portion of 7q based on the finding of an apparent hemizygous patient, phenotype Jk(a+b−), who should have been Jk(a+b+) and who also had a deletion of the long arm of chromosome 7. This assignment was strengthened by reports of a further association of the Colton blood group with monosomy of chromosome 7[17] and possible linkage of Kidd and Colton blood groups.[18] However, after reviewing 14 cases of patients with deletions of chromosome 7 Young et al[19] concluded in 1984 that the evidence for the placement of the Kidd gene on that portion of 7 was inadequate. Furthermore, Kidd had been tentatively assigned to chromosome 2 by its linkage with acid phosphatase (ACP1) and Colton blood groups.[20] An apparent linkage of insulin-dependent diabetes mellitus (IDDM) to Kidd was first reported in 1981 by Hodge and coworkers.[21] Since that report, additional studies by them[22] and other groups[23] have shown that there is no linkage to IDDM. The most recent discovery is that Kidd is on chromosome 18! Geitvik and coworkers[24] noted that it was linked to a restriction fragment polymorphism that was expressed whenever chromosome 18 was present in a cell hybrid. They also believe, based on other studies, that the *Kidd* locus must be in the portion of 18q11-p21.

The Kidd Antigens

Masouredis and coworkers[25] studied the number of Kidd antigen sites using ferritin labeling and found 11,300 ± 3100 sites in Jk^aJk^a individuals. One tempting explanation of the weakness of Kidd antibody reactions has always been that the number of sites may be inadequate for the limits of sensitivity of the antiglobulin test. This theory appears less likely in view of there being about 14,000 sites with which antibody can bind. The Kell antigen, K1, has only 3000 sites, which seems to be perfectly adequate for antibody detection.

The data on Kidd antigen-antibody reactions could support an alternative theory. Kidd antibodies are always capable of activating complement under appropriate conditions,[26 (p 659)] which should mean that the antigen sites are close enough together to allow IgG antibodies to form a doublet. Two molecules of IgG bound in close proximity form the complement activation site. Another important fact is that Kidd antibody

Table 3-2. Test Methodology

Method	Sensitivity	Comments
Saline antiglobulin	least	use fresh serum and test cells from homozygous individuals
Low-ionic stength saline, wash and additive	improved	may detect paraben-dependent anti-Kidd antibodies
Enzymes (2-stage)	equal to LISS	problems with false-positives
LIP[50]	variable	" " "
Manual Polybrene® [51]	variable	" " "
4% Ficin capillary[52]	variable	autoadsorb serum or dilute to avoid false positives
LIAHT[56]	best[55]	problems with false-positives
PEG[58]	very reliable[59]	do not read after 37 C incubation

reactivity is enhanced by a variety of techniques including enzymes, LISS and polyethylene glycol (PEG). These all involve a change in antibody-binding conditions that allows the antibody to get closer to the antigen site. Moreover, Kidd antigens are not denatured by enzymes, by enzymes plus sulphydryl reducing reagents, by chloroquine diphosphate or by 2-aminoethylisothiouronium bromide (AET) under conditions that readily alter other blood group antigens. It seems more likely that Kidd antigen sites may be clustered and not very accessible. Thus less antibody may be bound in tests that do not employ an antibody-enhancement technique. Whatever the reason, it is possible to enhance weak Kidd antibody reactions with methods listed in Table 3-2.

Kidd Antigens on Other Cell Lines

In 1974, Marsh, Øyen and Nichols[27] reported that Jk^a and Jk^b could not be detected on white cells by absorption tests but that anti-Jk3 was readily absorbed by the same cells. This claim has since been disputed by several studies that have shown that various cell lines do not demonstrate anti-Jk3 binding by fluorescence flow cytometry,[28] Staph protein A ^{125}I-SPA,[29] avidin-biotin complex immunoperoxidase staining[29] and two stage radioimmunoassay.[30] In justice to the earlier report, these sophisticated methods were not available then and the pitfalls of unexplained antibody loss in absorption methods are now widely recognized.

Kidd Antigen Alteration

McGinness, Leiberman, and Holland[31] reported an unusual case of autohemolysis in which a patient hemolyzed her red cells during episodes of *Proteus mirablis* bladder infection. The authors found that Jk(b−) cells could become reactive with anti-Jk^b after incubation with *P. mirablis* cultures. These workers have since found that *Streptococcus faecium* has similar properties.[32] Meyer and McGinniss[33] found that incubation of red cells with *Mycobacterium avium-intracellulare* cultures seemed to reduce the reactivity of Jk^a, Jk^b, S, s and U antigens on red cells. They studied this effect because sepsis with *M. avium-intracellulare* has become common in patients with acquired immune deficiency syndrome. Actual cases of antigen alterations must be very rare, but they show possibilities for the study of Kidd blood group biochemistry and potential advances in techniques.

Immune Response to Kidd Antigens

The antigens of the Kidd system are not very good immunogens compared with the Rh or K antigens. If 1000 Jk(a−) persons receive one dose of Jk(a+) blood, only seven will form the antibody.[34] Examples of pure anti-Jk^b are even rarer. However, if one looks at patients who have made more than one antibody, the incidence rises.[35] Mollison[36] noted that 20% of Jk(a−), Rh negative volunteers made anti-Jk^a plus anti-D if they were given Jk(a+), Rh positive blood. Anti-Jk^b also occurs more frequently in patients who make more than one antibody.

Kidd Antibodies

Although there is plenty of information about the in vivo behavior of Kidd antibodies in the literature, the data are somewhat biased by the number of reports of very difficult-to-detect Kidd antibodies and delayed hemolytic transfusion reactions. A consistent finding in immediate or delayed hemolytic transfusion reactions (HTR) caused by Kidd antibodies is the poor correlation between weak in vitro reactivity and severe in vivo hemolysis. The data point to Ig class, subclass and the ability to activate complement as being of greater clinical importance than antibody concentration and avidity. Several studies have shown that Kidd antibodies are almost always IgG of subclasses 1 and 3.[37,38] Occasionally IgM Kidd antibodies behave as saline agglutinins and are very valuable reagents.

Mollison[26(p 650)] includes the Kidd system in his discussion of antibodies that cause extravascular hemolysis. While most severe cases of HTR can have an intravascular phase with hemoglobinemia and hemoglobinuria, the commonest site of red cell destruction by Kidd antibodies is the liver. Although complement activation is a vital factor in intravascular hemolysis, Kidd antibodies activate complement differently than ABO antibodies. Large amounts of C4b2a3b (C5 convertase) need to be on a red cell for completion of the complement cascade.[39] If C3b is present as isolated fragments, direct hemolysis does not occur, but cell-bound IgG and C3b have a synergistic effect that causes rapid clearance in the liver. The rate of clearance varies from case to case. Incomplete clearance can be recognized in cases of delayed HTR in which adequate amounts of antibody are detected in the serum of patients with circulating incompatible red cells. Judd et al[40] in a prospective study of their patients with positive direct antiglobulin tests (DAT) found antibody in the serum of seven of 10 patients with anti-Jk^a in the eluate. Slower than expected clearance may be due to poor reticuloendothelial function or may be caused by inactivation of the red-cell-bound C3b to C3d, which makes the cells more resistant to lysis.

A serious problem is the rapid disappearance of Kidd antibodies. In some cases, the presence of Kidd antibodies may be so transient that the unfortunate patient has to experience several transfusion reactions before the cause is identified. The disappearance of Kidd antibodies does not seem to be a function of the patient's ability to maintain an immune response, since many patients who have Kidd antibodies that are no longer active have other strongly reactive, clinically significant antibodies. It is a rare patient indeed, like the one reported by Cox, McMican and Blumberg,[41] who had anti-Jk^b still detectable 16 years after it had first been identified.

It is important for blood bankers to be very careful in their criteria for identifying Kidd antibodies. The recommendation that whenever Kidd antibodies cannot be excluded, antigen-negative blood should be given, may have been justified 20 years ago but now seems unnecessarily conservative and wasteful.[42] Since these antibodies can be difficult to identify, especially in complex serological cases, enhancement techniques and appropriate criteria to define or exclude their presence are necessary. If a laboratory does not have the resources to perform the necessary tests it should refer the problem to one that does.

Hemolytic Disease of the Newborn (HDN)

Another aspect of the behavior of Kidd antibodies is their relatively mild affect on infants at risk for HDN. Unlike Rh system antibodies, hydrops fetalis or severe hemolysis requiring intrauterine or exchange transfusion is not expected. Some of the earliest reports describe severe cases of HDN but these were reported before the age of phototherapy and thus are hard to relate to current experience. In a review of 14 cases of maternal-fetal Kidd incompatibility,[43] only two infants needed exchange transfusion (both were before 1969). Walker[44] reported 30,000 obstetrical cases from his institution for the years 1979 to 1984. Only 41 mothers were at risk of HDN due to antibodies other than anti-D or ABO incompatibility. Of the 41, six cases were of anti-Jk^a in which five infants had no signs of HDN and one required phototherapy. The affected infant's bilirubin never rose above 12.9 mg/dl.

Anti-Jk3 is also not associated with severe HDN. Pierce et al[9] noted that it is usually detected in Jk(a−b−) mothers who have been transfused as opposed to having been sensitized only by pregnancy. They reported an interesting case of a Filipina woman who, during the delivery of her seventh child, was found to have anti-Jk3 plus anti-Jk^a. There were no records of any of her infants' having HDN, although after her second pregnancy she had received a transfusion. The infant had a positive DAT, and anti-Jk3 was recovered in the eluate. The infant's hemoglobin remained stable and his bilirubin never rose above 12.9 mg/dl. In a case reported by Kuczmarski, Bergen and Perkins,[45] a mother with an anti-Jk3 (titer 256) was studied; although rising titers and optical density values indicated potentially serious HDN, the infant only required phototherapy after induced delivery at 36 weeks.

Various factors may cause the weaker-than-expected hemolytic potential of Kidd antibodies during incompatible pregnancies. On the one hand, Kidd antibodies are known to be mostly IgG subclasses 1 and 3 and, therefore, should be readily transported across the placenta to react with the incompatible red cells. Also Kidd antigens are known to be well developed on the red cells of very young fetuses.[10(p 308)] Finally, the antibodies can bind complement, which should increase their hemolytic potential. However, the amount of antibody transported across the placenta is related to the titer, and most Kidd antibodies are not of high concentration. While Kidd antigens are well developed on fetal red cells, the dosage of antigen in an incompatible pregnancy must be that of a heterozygote. In vitro many Kidd antibodies react weakly or not at all with Jk(a+b+) red cells. Published reports of Kidd HDN make no mention of the presence of complement on the infants' cells. Kline[46] suggests that antibodies directed against antigens associated with integral functions of the red cells, such as Rh, may be more likely to cause severe HDN, although certainly the number of antigenic sites plays a role. The prediction of the severity of Kidd HDN must at present be evaluated by antibody titration and amniocentesis, if necessary. The usual mild course of HDN should make more drastic or elaborate intervention unnecessary.

In Vitro Behavior of Kidd Antibodies

One of the dilemmas in blood banking is how to detect all clinically significant antibodies using one standard technique. This is, of course, impossible and most approaches have the great drawback of detecting many unwanted positives and false positives. Failure to detect Kidd antibodies is a concern because they are a serious cause of immediate and delayed transfusion reactions. Yet efforts to increase sensitivity may overlook problems associated with false positives. Some of the methods listed in Table 3-2 are very effective in detecting weak Kidd antibodies, but are unsuitable for routine testing. However, when a Kidd antibody is suspected and routine methods of antibody identification have not given a clear-cut result, these more sensitive methods (with proper controls) can prove very useful.

The detection of weakly reactive Kidd antibodies is also an important part of the controversy about which antiglobulin (AHG) reagent should be used for compatibility testing. Proponents[47] of polyspecific antiglobulin sera have good data to support their assertion that dangerous Kidd antibodies will be missed unless the AHG reagent has both anti-IgG and anti-C3. Their concern becomes more valid if the crossmatch is abbreviated. More Kidd antibodies could be missed if the antibody screen were not performed with a polyspecific reagent.

On the other hand, the benefits of using anti-IgG AHG to avoid false positives are obvious and can eliminate much unnecessary testing. It seems (at least in some studies[48]) that complement-dependent Kidd antibodies are fairly rare. Perhaps enough data will become available to answer this question when enough laboratories have tried abbreviating the crossmatch.

Another problem with antiglobulin reagents is in their preparation. Manufacturers compare the dilutions of antiglobulin sera that give the best reactions with a number of antibodies in order to select the best dilution of the reagent. But as Mollison[26 (p 511)] points out, the best dilution for detecting anti-D antibodies is usually a weaker level of anti-IgG than that which reacts best with Kidd-antibody-coated cells. This may mean that the dilution of anti-IgG selected is not ideal for either but comes closer to an acceptable reaction for both. Issitt[49] also suggests that when selecting antiglobulin reagents one should compare titrations of Kidd and Duffy system antibodies because these seem to show a greater variability between lots than Rh antibodies.

Selection of Test Method

The methods listed in Table 3-2 include both standard procedures and some that are newly described, whose disadvantages are not yet known. In a particular case any one procedure may prove to be more effective than another in detecting unusual Kidd antibodies. Techniques that do not require the antiglobulin test may give more reliable reactions with Kidd antibodies of poor affinity that may not stay bound during the washing phase. Examples of these are the LIP[50], manual Polybrene®[51] and 4% ficin[52] tests. Kidd antibodies have been described that were detectable only by these methods.[53]

Steane et al[54] proposed a manual Polybrene® crossmatch as a suitable alternative to dropping the antiglobulin phase of the crossmatch, because of the test's ability to detect clinically significant antibodies, including those of the Kidd system. Postoway and Garratty[55] recently evaluated a low-ionic test method[56] that also used a low-ionic antiglobulin reagent. They found that many antibodies, including those of the Kidd system, reacted best by this method. Unfortunately the problem of false positives was so great that they suggested this method be used for special situations when antibodies cannot be demonstrated by routine techniques.

Enzyme techniques, particularly two-stage methods, are very useful for working with Kidd antibodies. In the author's laboratory, it is not uncommon for a weak Kidd antibody that reacts only with cells from donors who are homozygous, to react strongly with enzyme-treated Jk(a+b+) cells. While it is possible for a Kidd antibody not to react as well or better with enzyme-treated cells, such a reaction should be viewed with suspicion. A bizarre phenomenon involving enzyme-treated red cells was reported by Lown et al[57] who found two examples of anti-Jk^a that inhibited the agglutination of enzyme-treated cells by Rh antibodies. The effect was eliminated if EDTA was added to the test sera. The authors thought the enzyme test results could be misinterpreted if sera with multiple antibodies had this problem. The ability of Kidd antibodies to hemolyze enzyme-treated incompatible red cells is well known. If the red cells are suspended in an Alsevers-type diluent, hemolysis almost never occurs (personal observation).

The polyethylene glycol (PEG) method described by Nance and Garratty[58] has also been shown to be effective in enhancing weakly reactive Kidd antibodies.[59] The PEG method has the added advantage of not enhancing some of the clinically insignificant antibodies such as those of high titre, low avidity (HTLA). This could prove useful in eliminating or confirming the presence of Kidd antibodies in sera with HTLA antibodies.

The Kidd System and Autoantibodies

Kidd antibodies very rarely cause warm autoimmune hemolytic anemia (WAIHA), but all three specificities have been described (Table 3-3).[60-71] Issitt et al[63] used absorption studies with Jk(a−b−) cells to determine whether auto-anti-Jk3 was a common component of anti-dl warm autoantibodies. Although they found one example of an auto-anti-Jk^a the other 34 anti-dl sera they examined did not contain auto-Kidd antibodies. In some cases the autoantibody is associated with an infectious process but anti-Jk^a has also been seen in a patient taking α-methyldopa[62] and another taking chlorpropamide.[67] (See Chapter 4.) There have also been reports of benign Kidd autoantibodies[61, 63, 71] and one unusual case, in which the apparent auto-anti-Jk3 plus anti-Jk^b was really a mimicking antibody that could be completely absorbed by Jk(a−b−) red cells.[65] This "mimicking" antibody merely showed a preference for Jk-positive red cells and caused mild hemolysis.

Obarski et al[70] studied a Jk(a+b−) patient with a transient suppression of her Kidd phenotype. The patient typed as

THE KIDD BLOOD GROUP SYSTEM 65

Table 3-3. Kidd Autoantibodies

Specificity	Hemolysis?	Association?	Patient History and Comments
Anti-Jk^a	yes		40-yr-old female, pernicious anemia[60]
Anti-Jk^a	no		17-yr-old female, healthy donor[61]
Anti-Jk^a	yes	Aldomet	53-yr-old female, hypertension[62]
Anti-Jk^b	yes	P. mirablis infection	female, nephrectomy, persistent[31] bladder infections
Anti-Jk^a	no		27-yr-old female, pregnant DAT persisted for 2 years[63] female[64]
Anti-Jk^a	yes		25-yr-old female, pregnant[65]
Anti-Jk^b + and anti-Jk3	mild		
Anti-Jk^a	yes	Legionella pneumonia	44-yr-old male[66]
Anti-Jk^a	yes	Chlorpropamide	43-yr-old female, hypoglycemic[67]
Anti-Jk^a	yes	Fever, unknown origin	8-month-old female[68]
Anti-Jk^a	yes		45-yr-old male[69]
Anti-Jk3	yes		86-yr-old female, myelofibrosis[70]
Anti-Jk3	no	Evans syndrome	31-yr-old female, pregnant[71]

Jk(a−b−) and had an anti-Jk3 that necessitated transfusing her with Jk(a−b−) blood.

Conclusion

The literature offers a wealth of information about the Kidd system, especially its association with transfusion reactions. Because of their unusual properties Kidd antibodies should be useful for studying new reagents and new methods of antibody detection. Whether crossmatch procedures will ever be improved to the point that delayed transfusion reactions can be avoided is impossible to predict, but it seems unlikely. Finally, recent advances in the purification of the Kidd antigen and studies of the 2M-urea effect on Jk(a−b−) red cells signal that a significant era in our understanding of this blood group is about to begin.

References

1. Allen FH, Diamond LK, Niedziela B. A new blood group antigen. Nature 1951;167:482.
2. Plaut G, Ikin EW, Mourant AE, Sanger R, Race RR. A new blood group antibody, anti-Jk^b. Nature 1953;171:431.
3. Pinkerton FJ, Mermod LE, Liles BA, Jack JA, Noades J. The phenotype Jk(a−b−) in the Kidd blood group system. Vox Sang 1959;4:155-60.
4. Dykes D. The use of frequency tables in parentage testing. In: Silver H, ed. Probability of inclusion in paternity testing. Arlington, VA: American Association of Blood Banks, 1982:15-44.
5. Grunbaum BW, Selvin S, Myhre BA, Pace N. Distribution of gene frequencies and discrimination probabilities for 22 human blood genetic systems in four racial groups. J Forensic Sci 1980;25:428-44.
6. Woodfield DG, Douglas R, Smith J, Simpson A, Pinder L, Stavely JM. The Jk(a−b−) phenotype in New Zealand Polynesians. Transfusion 1982;22:276-8.
7. Okubo Y, Yamaguchi H, Nagao N, Tomita T, Seno T, Tanaka M. Heterogeneity of the phenotype Jk(a−b−) found in Japanese. Transfusion 1986;26:237-9.
8. Humphrey AJ, Morel PA. Further evidence of heterogeneity within the Kidd blood group system. Transfusion 1976;16:242-4.

9. Pierce SR, Hardman JT, Steele S, Beck ML. Hemolytic disease of the newborn associated with anti-Jk3. Transfusion 1980;20:189-91.
10. Issitt PD. Applied blood group serology. 3rd ed. Miami: Montgomery Scientific, 1985.
11. Day D, Perkins HA, Sams B. The minus-minus phenotype in the Kidd system. Transfusion 1965;5:315-9.
12. Habibi B, Avril J, Fouillade MT, Lopez M, Vaucelle R, Salmon C. Jk(a−b−) phenotype in a French family. Quantitative evidence for the inheritance of a silent allele (Jk). Hematologia 1976;10:403-6.
13. Heaton DC, McLoughlin K. Jk(a−b−) red blood cells resist urea lysis. Transfusion 1982;22:70-1.
14. Crawford MN, Greenwalt TJ, Sasaki T, Tippett P, Sanger R, Race RR. The phenotype Lu(a−b−) together with unconventional Kidd groups in one family. Transfusion 1961;1:228-32.
15. Arcara PC, O'Connor MA, Dimmette RM. A family with three Jk(a−b−) members (abstract). Transfusion 1969;9:282.
16. Shokeir MHK, Ying KL, Pabello P. Deletion of the long arm of chromosome no. 7: tentative assignment of the Kidd (Jk) locus. Clin Genet 1973;4:360-8.
17. de la Chapelle A, Vuopio P, Sanger R, Teesdale PH. Monosomy 7 and the Colton blood groups. Lancet 1975;2:817.
18. Mohr J, Eiberg H. Colton blood groups: indication of linkage with the Kidd (Jk) system as support for assignment to chromosome 7. Clin Genet 1977;11:372-4.
19. Young RS, Weaver DD, Kukolich MK, et al. Terminal and interstitial deletions of the long arm of chromosome 7: a review with five new cases. Am J Med Genet 1984;17:437-50.
20. Lewis M, Kaita H, Philipps S, Steinberg AG, Giblett ER, Anderson JE. Analysis of linkage relationships of Co, Jk, and K with each other and with chromosome 2 loci ACP1 and Km. Ann Hum Genet 1982;46:349-54.
21. Hodge HE, Anderson CE, Neiswanger K, et al. Close genetic linkage between diabetes mellitus and Kidd blood group. Lancet 1981;2:893-5.
22. Hodge SE, Anderson CE, Neiswanger K, et al. Association studies between type 1 (insulin-dependent) diabetes and 27 genetic markers: lack of association between type 1 diabetes and Kidd blood group. Diabetologia 1983;25:343-7.

23. Dunsworth TS, Rich SS, Swanson J, Barbosa J. No evidence for linkage analysis between diabetes and the Kidd marker. Diabetes 1982;31:991-3.
24. Geitvik GA, Høyheim B, Gedde-Dahl T, et al. The Kidd (JK) blood group locus assigned to chromosome 18 by close linkage to a DNA-RFLP. Hum Genet 1987;77:205-9.
25. Masouredis SP, Sudora E, Mahan L, Victoria EJ. Quantitative immunoferritin microscopy of Fy^a, Fy^b, Jk^a, U, and Di^b antigen site numbers on human red cells. Blood 1980;56:969-77.
26. Mollison PL. Blood transfusion in clinical medicine. 7th ed. Oxford: Blackwell Scientific, 1983.
27. Marsh WL, Øyen R, Nichols ME. Kidd-blood group antigens of leukocytes and platelets. Transfusion 1974;14:378-81.
28. Dunstan RA. Status of major red cell blood group antigens on neutrophils, lymphocytes, and monocytes. Br J Haematol 1986;62:301-9.
29. Gaidulis L, Branch DR, Lazar GS, Petz LD, Blume KG. The red cell antigens A, B, D, U, Ge, Jk3, and Yt^a. Br J Haematol 1985;60:659-68.
30. Dunstan RA, Simpson MB, Rosse WF. Erythrocyte antigens on human platelets. Absence of Rh, Duffy, Kell, Kidd, and Lutheran antigens. Transfusion 1984;24:243-6.
31. McGinniss MH, Leiberman R, Holland PV. The Jk^b red cell antigen and gram negative organisms (abstract). Transfusion 1979;19:663.
32. McGinniss MG, MacLowry JD, Holland PV. Acquisition of Kell-like antigen by Kell negative red cells (abstract). Transfusion 1978;18:624.
33. Meyer MT, McGinniss MH. Changes in red cell antigen expression following exposure to *Mycobacterium avium-intracellulare* (abstract). Transfusion 1985;25:446.
34. Toy PTC, Vyas GN. Blood transfusion reactions. In: Englefriet CP, van Loghem JJ, von dem Borne AEGK, eds. Immunohaematology. Amsterdam: Elsevier Science, 1984:130.
35. Mollison PL. Red cell destruction in vivo by alloantibodies. In: Mohn JF, Plunkett RW, Cunningham RK, Lambert RM, eds. Human blood groups. Basel: S Karger, 1977:65-74.
36. Mollison PL. Rh immunization and its suppression. In: Schmidt PF, ed. Progress in transfusion and transplan-

tation. Washington, DC: American Association of Blood Banks, 1972;119-33.
37. Szymanski IO, Huff SR, Delsignore R. An autoanalyzer test to determine immunoglobulin class and IgG subclass of blood group antibodies. Transfusion 1982;22: 90-5.
38. Hardman JT, Beck ML. Hemagglutination in capillaries: correlation with blood group specificity and IgG subclass. Transfusion 1981;21:343-6.
39. Davey RJ. Mechanisms of premature red cell destruction. In: Judd WJ, Barnes A, eds. Clinical and serological aspects of transfusion reactions. Arlington, VA: American Association of Blood Banks, 1982:8.
40. Judd WJ, Butch SH, Oberman HA, Steiner EA, Bauer RC. The evaluation of a positive direct antiglobulin test in pretransfusion testing. Transfusion 1980;20:17-23.
41. Cox MT, McMican A, Blumberg N. Case report of an anti-Jk^b persisting for sixteen years (letter). Transfusion 1983;23:362.
42. Salmon C, Cartron JP, Rouger P. The human blood groups. New York: Masson Publishing, 1984:256-8.
43. Dorner I, Moore JA, Chaplin H. Combined maternal erythrocyte autosensitization and materno-fetal Jk^a incompatibility. Transfusion 1974;14:211-9.
44. Walker RH. Relevancy in selection of serological tests for the obstetrical patient. In: Garratty G, ed. Hemolytic disease of the newborn. Arlington, VA: American Association of Blood Banks, 1984:173-203.
45. Kuczmarski CA, Bergren MO, Perkins HA. Mild hemolytic disease of the newborn due to anti-Jk3: a serological study of the family's Kidd antigens. Vox Sang 1982;43: 340-4.
46. Kline WE. The chemistry of blood group antigens and antibodies in hemolytic disease of the newborn. In: Bell CA, ed. A seminar on perinatal blood banking. Washington, DC: American Association of Blood Banks, 1978:1-25.
47. Howell P, Giles CM. A detailed serological study of five anti-Jk^a sera reacting by the antiglobulin technique. Vox Sang 1983;45:129-38.
48. Petz LD, Garratty G. Antiglobulin sera—past, present and future. Transfusion 1978;18:257-68.
49. Issitt PD. Evaluation of antiglobulin reagents. In: Myhre BA, ed. A seminar on performance evaluation. Washing-

ton, DC: American Association of Blood Banks, 1976:25-74.
50. Rosenfield RE, Shaikh SH, Inella F, Kaczera Z, Kochwa S. Augmentation of hemagglutination by low ionic conditions. Transfusion 1979;19:499-510.
51. Lalezari P, Jiang AF. The manual Polybrene test: a simple and rapid procedure for detection of red cell antibodies. Transfusion 1980;20:206-11.
52. Hardman JT, Pierce SR, Crawford MN, Beck ML. A modified capillary test using 4% ficin. Transfusion 1981; 21:330-1.
53. Garratty G, Vengelen-Tyler V, Postoway N, Brunt D, Nance S, Schulman I. Hemolytic transfusion reactions (HTR) associated with antibodies not detectable by routine procedures (abstract). Transfusion 1982;22:429.
54. Steane EA, Steane SM, Montgomery SR, Pearson JR. A proposal for compatibility testing incorporating the manual hexadimethrine bromide (Polybrene) test. Transfusion 1985;25:540-4.
55. Postoway N, Garratty G. Evaluation of a newly described low ionic antiglobulin test (abstract). Transfusion 1987; 27:314.
56. Ahn JH, Rosenfield RE, Kochwa S. Low ionic antiglobulin tests. Transfusion 1987;27:125-33.
57. Lown JA, Holland PA, Barr AL. Inhibition of serological reactions with enzyme treated red cells by complement binding alloantibodies. Vox Sang 1984;46:300-5.
58. Nance S, Garratty G. Polyethylene glycol: A new potentiator of red blood cell antigen-antibody reactions. Am J Clin Pathol 1987;87:633-5.
59. Vengelen-Tyler V, Choy C. A comparative study of antibody enhancement techniques (abstract). Transfusion 1986;26:570.
60. van Loghem JJ, van der Hart M. Varieties of specific autoantibodies in acquired haemolytic anaemia. Vox Sang 1954;4:2-11.
61. Holmes LD, Pierce SR, Beck M. Autoanti-Jk^a in a healthy blood donor (abstract). Transfusion 1976;16:521.
62. Patten E, Beck CE, Scholl C, Stroope RA, Wukasch C. Autoimmune hemolytic anemia with anti-Jk^a specificity in a patient taking Aldomet. Transfusion 1977;17:517-20.
63. Issitt PD, Pavone BG, Frohlich JA, McGuire Mallory D. Absence of auto anti-Jk3 as a component of anti-dl. Transfusion 1980;20:733-6.

64. Judd WJ, Steiner EA, Cochran RK. Paraben-associated autoanti-Jk^a antibodies. Transfusion 1982;22:31-5.
65. Ellisor SS, Reid ME, O'Day T, Swanson J, Papenfus L, Avoy DR. Autoantibodies mimicking anti-Jk^b plus anti-Jk3 associated with autoimmune hemolytic anemia in a primipara who delivered an unaffected infant. Vox Sang 1983;45:53-9.
66. Strikas R, Seifert MR, Lentino JR. Autoimmune hemolytic anemia and *Legionella pneumophila* pneumonia. Ann Intern Med 1983;99:345.
67. Sosler SD, Behzad O, Garratty G, Lee CL, Postoway N, Khuomo O. Acute hemolytic anemia associated with a chlorpropamide-induced apparent auto anti-Jk^a. Transfusion 1984;24:206-9.
68. Sander RP, Hardy NM, Van Meter SA. Anti-Jk^a autoimmune hemolytic anemia in an infant. Transfusion 1987;27:58-60.
69. Ciaffoni S, Ferro I, Potenza R, Campo G. Evans syndrome: a case of autoimmune thrombocytopenia and autoimmune hemolytic anemia caused by anti-Jk^a. Haematologica 1987;72:245-7.
70. Obarski G, Hartnett PL, Prewitt PL, Issitt PD. The Jk(a−b−) phenotype, probably occurring as a transient phenomenon (abstract). Transfusion 1987;27:548.
71. O'Day T. A second example of auto anti-Jk3 (letter). Transfusion 1987;27:442.

In: Pierce, SR, and Macpherson, CR, eds.
Blood Group Systems: Duffy, Kidd and Lutheran
Arlington, VA: American Association
of Blood Banks, 1988

4

The Kidd Blood Group System: Drug-Related Antibodies and Biochemistry

JoAnn Edwards-Moulds, MS, MT(ASCP)SBB

BLOOD GROUP SEROLOGISTS HAVE historically played important roles in detecting and identifying rare or unusual blood group phenotypes and antibodies. However, more recent advances in the investigation of red cell blood groups have been in the areas of membrane biochemistry and gene cloning. Although such work is only just emerging for the Kidd blood group, it too holds promise of increasing our understanding of blood group structure and function.

Chemical and Drug-Related Antibodies

Drug-Related Antibodies

As discussed in Chapter 3, Kidd antibodies can be implicated in warm autoimmune hemolytic anemia (AIHA). Only one case of chlorpropamide-induced AIHA has been reported[1] which had Jk^a specificity. An earlier example of chlorpropamide-induced anemia had no reported blood group specificity;[2] the two nonreactive cells in this case were later typed as $Jk(a+)$,[1] excluding that specificity. In both cases the patients had an acute hemolytic crisis when taking the hypoglycemic drug chlorpropamide.

The Jk^a specificity in the case of Sosler et al[1] could be demonstrated only when the drug was present in the test system, thus the authors' term "apparent auto-anti-Jk^a."[1] The antibody cross-reacted with three other sulfonylureas:

JoAnn Edwards-Moulds, MS, MT(ASCP)SBB, PhD Candidate, Division of Rheumatology and Clinical Immunogenetics, University of Texas Health Science Center, Houston, Texas

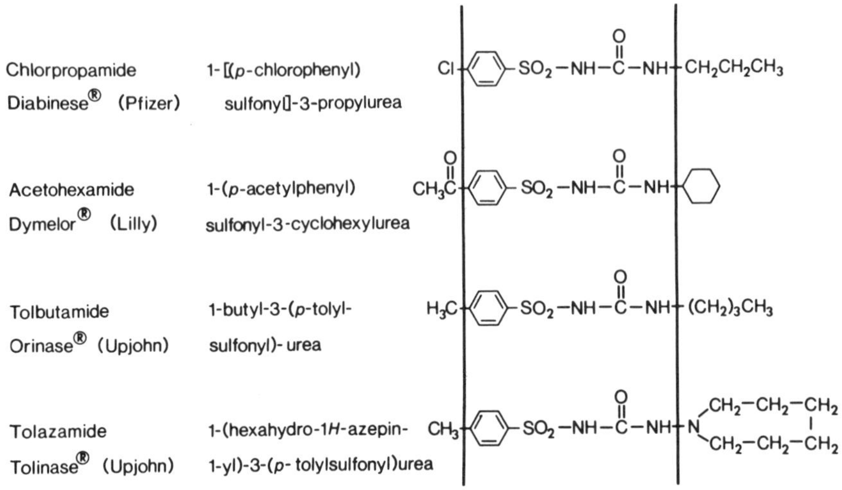

Figure 4-1. Chemical similarities of the four drugs that react with an apparent auto-anti-Jk^a. (Reprinted with permission.[1])

acetamide, tolbutamide and tolazamide. Bird et al[3] had previously described a case of tolbutamide-associated AIHA in which the antibody cross-reacted with chlorpropamide-treated red cells. It is interesting to note that each of these drugs contains a urea structure (Fig 4-1); as discussed below, urea plays a key role in the identification of the Jk(a−b−) phenotype.

LISS-Related Antibodies: Parabens

In addition to the Kidd autoantibodies that cause increased cell destruction (see Chapter 3), several examples of benign auto-anti-Jk^a have been reported. Most of these appeared after commercial low ionic strength solutions (LISS) came into routine use for antibody screening tests. Since reports of antibodies to reagent additives (including antibiotics, dyes, EDTA, sodium caprylate and others[4]) are numerous it is not unusual that another additive should be incriminated.

Halima et al[5] described a 60-year-old Caucasian male diagnosed postoperatively as having Crohn's disease. During compatibility testing, a strongly reactive anti-Jk^a was detected using LISS-suspended red cells that was not detected in saline or albumin. Unexpectedly, the patient's autocontrol was positive when using his LISS-suspended red cells, yet a direct antiglobulin test and eluate were negative. His red cells typed as Jk(a+b+). Identical results were reported by Judd et al[6] in two of three patients with paraben-associated anti-Jk^a.

These antibodies seemed similar to the chlorpropamide antibody reported by Logue et al[2] in that they reacted in vitro only in the presence of the drug or chemical. Both reactions involved immune complexes and the activation of complement that was detected by anti-C3 reagents. Two of the LISS-Jk[a] antibodies also caused direct agglutination of red cells suspended in LISS plus paraben. Unlike the chlorpropamide antibodies which caused rapid hemolysis, the LISS-dependent anti-Jk[a] caused no overt signs of hemolytic anemia. Judd et al's patients all had normal reticulocyte counts and hemoglobin levels.[6] Thus, both papers concluded that these types of antibodies had no clinical significance.

By dissecting and testing the individual components of the commercial LISS solutions, both groups of investigators found that the additive methylparaben caused the unusual serologic reactivity. Propyl- and methylparaben were used as preservatives in the two of six commercial LISS preparations that gave positive reactions. The only other reactive chemical tested by Halima et al[5] was methylsalicylate (wintergreen). Judd and coworkers[6] tested a large number of chemicals for reactivity with serum from their three patients and found several other compounds that could demonstrate the anti-Jk[a]. The combined results of these two groups of researchers are shown in Table 4-1. There are some discrepancies between the two groups and indeed in one study not all of the samples reacted with all of the reagents tested. This could be due to a difference in concentration, pH or other qualitative factors.

Halima et al[5] found their patient's antibody to have a narrow chemical specificity, reacting only with methyl esters of hydroxybenzoic acid when the hydroxyl groups were in the para or ortho positions. They speculated that when the hydroxyl group was in either position it could donate electrons to increase the electron density of the carbon atom in the benzene ring where the methyl group was attached. Their results suggested that hydrogen bonding may be important in the antibody's reacting with its epitope. Judd et al[6] concluded that the antibodies were dependent upon aromatic compounds (eg, benzene ring) and noted that hydroxyl groups were present on all reactive compounds. They hypothesized that the Jk[a] antigen was structurally altered in the presence of these chemicals making it reactive with antibodies (anti-Jk[a]) in the sera tested. This, however, does not explain why all four patients tested and phenotyped as Jk(a+b+) would preferentially produce auto-anti-Jk[a].

Table 4-1. Chemical Compounds Tested for Apparent Anti-Jk^a Specificity[5,6]

Reactive	Nonreactive	Equivocal
benzyl alcohol	aniline	dimethyl phthalate
butylparaben	anisole	ethylparaben*
dibutyl phthalate	benzene	phenol
methylparaben	benzoic acid	propylparaben*
methylsalicylate	m-butyl-B-D-glucoside	
2-phenoxyethanol	t-butyl-B-D-glucoside	
	chloramphenicol	
	p-chloromercuribenzoate	
	chlorpropamide	
	cyclohexanone	
	diethyl stilbestrol	
	Dilantin®	
	dipotassium EDTA	
	ethyl alcohol	
	m-ethylphenyl-B-D-glucoside	
	m-hydroxybenzoate	
	o-hydroxybenzoate	
	p-hydroxybenzoate	
	m-isopropylphenyl-B-D-glucoside	
	p-methoxybenzoate	
	methylacetoacetate	
	methylanthranilate	
	methylnicotinate	
	phenylalanine	
	salicin	
	sodium azide	
	sodium benzoate	
	sodium caprylate	
	thimerosal	
	tyrosine	

*Not all patients from same study showed reactivity

The etiology of paraben-associated anti-Jk^a is unknown. The stimulus may be viral or bacterial since all four patients had a recent history of such infection prior to the appearance of the antibody. The paraben-related substances are also widely used in cosmetics, food preservation and pharmaceuticals, and this may be the source of antibody stimulation. Clearly, the story is not complete concerning paraben-associated anti-Jk^a. Some important facts, however, should be remembered: 1) these antibodies do not react with all LISS products—only those containing paraben or other implicated additives; 2) they are not anti-Jk^a antibodies—they are antibodies that react with the appropriate chemical to form immune complexes that preferentially bind Jk(a+) red cells; and 3) as such, they are not true autoantibodies and are of doubtful clinical significance. Although two of the patients reported did receive Jk(a−) blood as a precaution, this is probably not necessary if the patient can be accurately phenotyped as Jk(a+).

Biochemistry of the Kidd Antigens

Number and Location

Little information has been published concerning the biochemistry of the Kidd blood group antigens. The weak reactions observed with many examples of anti-Jk^a were thought, early on, to be due to a small number of antigen binding sites on the red cell. However, in 1980, Masouredis et al[7] reported the use of immunoferritin microscopy to quantitate red cell antigen number. They found 11,300 ± 3100 sites on Jk^aJk^a red cells but only 1100 ± 370 sites on Jk^bJk^b cells. One may conclude that since these numbers are comparable to estimates for KK or Fy^aFy^b the weak reactions are not due to decreased receptor binding sites. However, the authors point out that the findings with ghost membranes may not reflect the antigen arrangement of intact red cell membranes.

Many blood group antigens are found in locations other than the red cell. There is currently no evidence that "Kidd substance" is found in plasma, urine, saliva, human milk or other fluids. In 1974, Marsh et al[8] found that neutrophils had strong absorptive capacity for anti-Jk^{a}Jk^b (-Jk3) but did not absorb individual examples of anti-Jk^a or -Jk^b. They also found that Jk3 was not present on lymphocytes and platelets. Several subsequent studies[9-11] using more sophisticated techniques have not found Jk^a, Jk^b or Jk3 present on neutrophils, lymphocytes or monocytes, nor Jk^a and Jk^b on platelets. Three examples of anti-Jk3 were tested for lymphocytotoxicity activity and were negative.[8] Habibi et al[12] tested the sera from two Jk(a−b−) donors who both had anti-Jk3 and could not demonstrate any lymphocytotoxicity or complement-fixing antiplatelet activity. Both leukocytes and platelets from the Jk(a−b−) donors also failed to absorb two other examples of anti-Jk3.

Biochemistry

A report[13] presented at the 1979 meeting of the American Association of Blood Banks described a hemolytic transfusion reaction due to an anti-Jk^b which was later[14] shown to be an autoantibody. Since the patient had chronic urinary tract infections due to a species of *Proteus*, *Proteus mirabilis* was studied for Jk^b-like activity. When red cells were incubated with *P. mirabilis*, *Micrococcus* or *Streptococcus faecium*[14] they became agglutinable by anti-Jk^b. Although these reports have not led to any definitive biochemical answers, they are intriguing, especially in light of bacterial associations with other blood group antigens.

Some information, however, is beginning to emerge concerning the Kidd antigens. Because antigen reactivity was destroyed by heating red cells at 56 C for 5 minutes, it was thought that Kidd may be protein in nature.[15] Several investigators have studied red cell membrane proteins from various Jk(a−b−) donors using sodium dodecyl sulfate-polyacrylamide gel electrophoresis (SDS-PAGE). No significant abnormalities have been noted[15,16]; however, this type of electrophoresis cannot detect all changes in the membrane.

Okubo et al[16] used PAGE in the absence of SDS to study two Jk(a−b−) donors of the suppressor type [*In(Jk)*] and four donors of the amorph type (*JkJk*). They observed two additional bands not seen in normal controls. A band was distinctly present at the 67-kD position in both the *In(Jk)* and the *JkJk* membrane preparations (Fig 4-2).

In another approach, Sinor et al[17] used a dot-blot method in attempts to isolate the Kidd protein. Red cells of varying Kidd phenotype were sensitized with anti-Jk^a, -Jk^b or -Jk3 and layered onto nylon membranes containing immobilized anti-human IgG. Eluates were prepared and analyzed by SDS-PAGE. Their results suggested that a 45-kD protein may carry the Kidd blood group antigens.

Urea Lysis Phenomenon

Pinkerton et al[18] first reported the Jk(a−b−) phenotype in a Filipina and postulated a third allele named *Jk*. Crawford and colleagues[19] gave evidence that the *Jk* gene existed in the Caucasian population. Although of highest frequency in

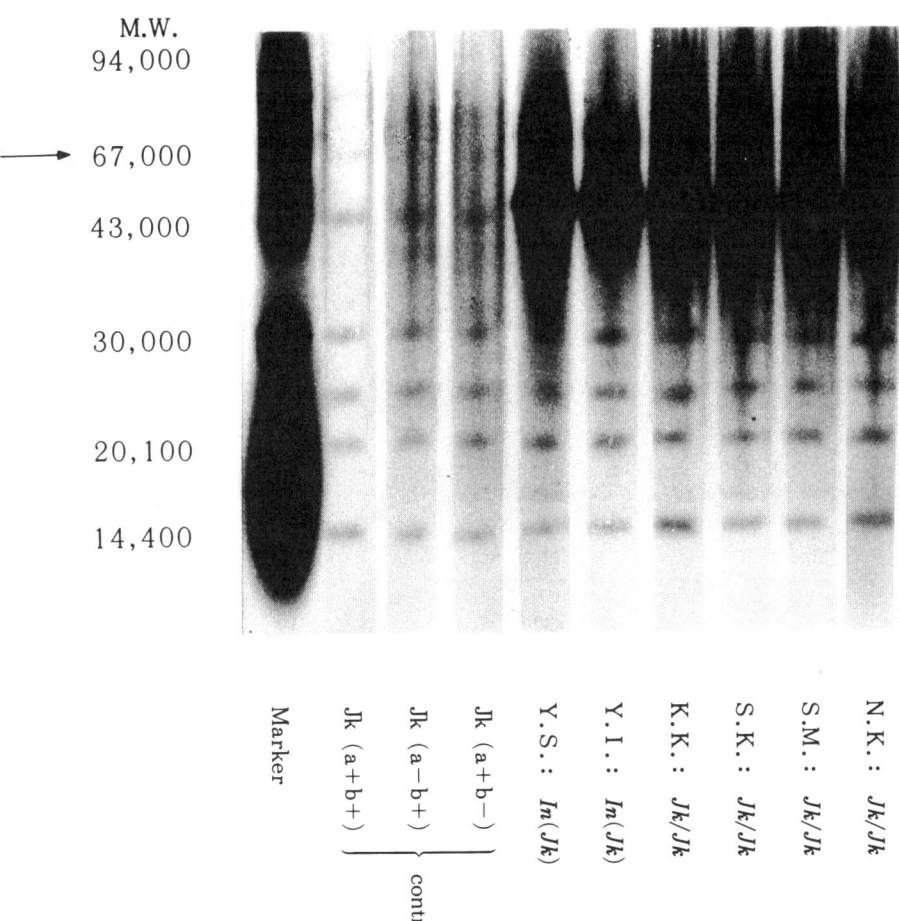

Figure 4-2. Polyacrylamide gel electrophoresis of red cell membrane proteins from *In(Jk)* and *JkJk* donors. (Reprinted with permission.[16])

Polynesians,[20, 21] several examples of the Jk(a−b−) phenotype in Caucasians have now been reported.[12, 22-24] The Jk(a−b−) phenotype in Japanese due to a suppressor gene was reported by Okubo et al.[16] In addition, an example of a transient Jk(a−b−) was recently reported by Obarski et al.[25]

The Jk(a−b−) phenotype has proven invaluable in the investigation of the structure and function of the Kidd antigens. A key paper by Heaton and McLoughlin[26] renewed interest in this null phenotype. While testing a patient diagnosed as having aplastic anemia, they found unexpectedly high automated platelet counts which were below normal when

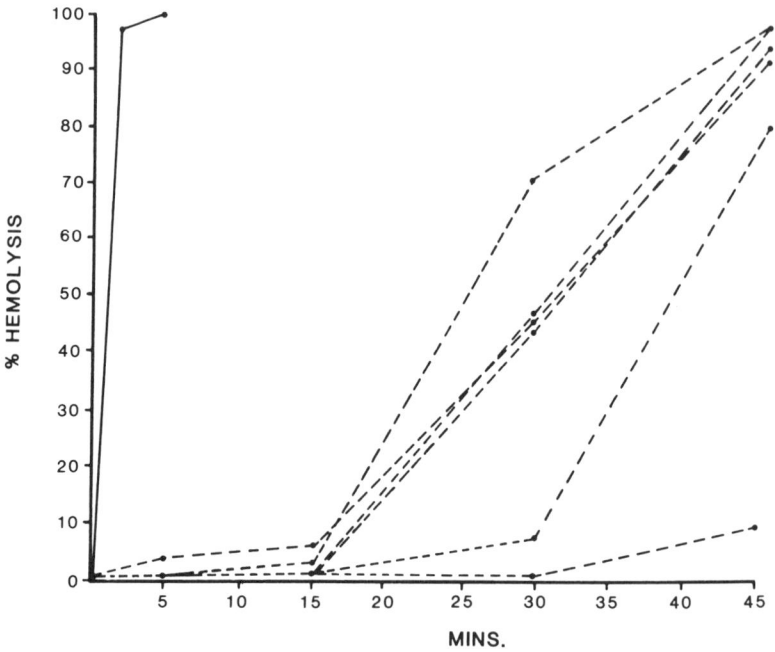

Figure 4-3. Lytic time curves of normal and Jk(a−b−) red cells suspended in 2M aqueous urea. Normal = solid line, Jk(a−b−) = dashed lines.

tested manually. Further investigation revealed that the elevated counts were due to red cells remaining unlysed in the lytic agent, 2M urea. Resistance to urea lysis has since been adapted and automated for screening of blood donors by several blood centers.[16, 27, 28]

In studying the urea lysis phenomenon, several researchers have found that the Jk(a−b−) red cells do not totally resist lysis but rather delay lysis for 15-30 minutes (see Fig 4-3).[26, 28, 29] In the Japanese report,[16] the optical densities obtained with hemolysates from In(Jk) red cells were higher than those from JkJk cells. However, it is difficult to compare these results as they were not normalized for hemoglobin content of the red cells.

Jk(a−b−) red cells have been tested with a battery of known lytic agents to study their unusual lytic properties in urea.[29, 30] Reagents tested to date have included: polyhydroxyl alcohols—glycerol, propylene glycol, ethylene glycol; detergents—cetyltrimethylammnonium bromide, sodium dodecyl sulphate, Triton X, Brij-35, digitonin, saponin, melittin; enzymes—phospholipase C-I and C-III, streptolysin O; and urea-related reagents—thiourea, methylurea, formamide, acetamide, quinidine hydrochloride. Each group of reagents causes lysis by a slightly different mechanism. The detergent group causes the membrane to fragment and solubilize while the enzymes usually act by hydrolyzing membrane lipids. One subset of the lytic agents is the channel formers (melittin and streptolysin) which cause pores to open in the membrane somewhat like the complement cascade. It is also possible to place digitonin and saponin in a separate category as they specifically interact with membrane cholesterol to cause lysis. The Jk(a−b−) red cells exhibited normal lytic curves when tested with all these lytic agents (with the exception of urea and methylurea).[29,30]

The mechanism of urea lysis in normal red cells is not due to its protein-denaturing capabilities. Urea and related compounds, such as thiourea,[31] move across the cell membrane and cause osmotic imbalances. Although there is still some conflict as to whether this occurs through a pore or by a specialized transport protein, the end result is the same. Reports by Jay and Rowlands[32] and Sha'afi et al[33] indicate that entrance of a permeant such as urea into the red cell causes an influx of water and cell lysis. The rate of red cell swelling depends not only on the membrane permeability to the solute but also to the osmotic gradient.[32]

Therefore, addition of salts to the aqueous urea should counterbalance osmotic lysis. This is what was observed when normal red cells were tested with 2M urea prepared in 0.4% or 0.8% phosphate buffered saline (PBS) and 0.15M citrate buffer.[34] In 2M urea/0.4% PBS an average of 50% lysis at 5 minutes was observed for normal red cells. Interestingly, four samples from donors known to be *Jk* heterozygotes exhibited lytic rates intermediate between normals and nulls (see Fig 4-4).[35] When suspended in 2M urea prepared in isosmotic buffers, the normal cells gave essentially no lysis for test periods up to 60 minutes.[24] Thus, urea alone could not be causing the hemolysis as the concentration of urea was equal in all reagents.

Transport Studies

The red cell possesses a semipermeable membrane through which water and solutes flow. Some substances can simply diffuse through the lipid bilayer while others must be actively transported (eg, Na^+/K^+). Although water can enter the red cell by diffusion, only 10% of water movement takes place in this manner.[36] There is considerable evidence that the bulk

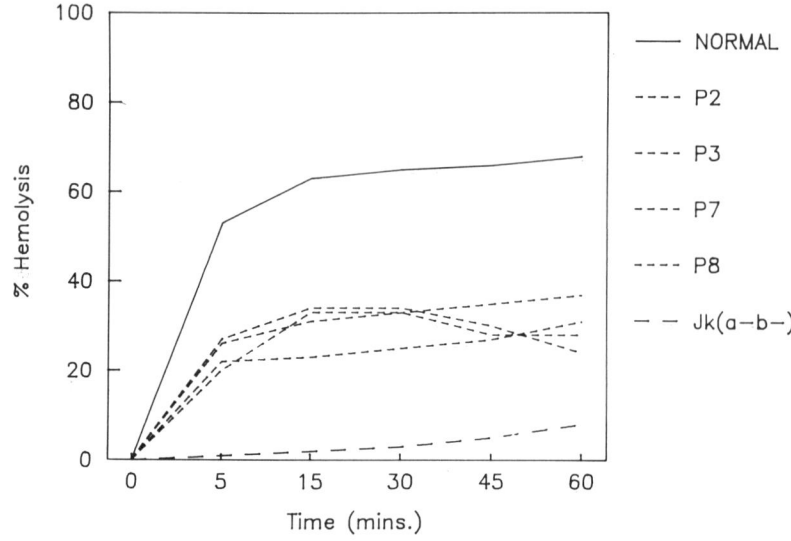

Figure 4-4. Lytic time curves of four *Jk* heterozygous red cells (P2, 3, 7, 8) suspended in 2M urea/0.4% PBS compared to average normal and average Jk(a−b−) curves.

of water moves through polar pores or water channels.[37-39] These pores are composed of membrane proteins that are positively charged in the area lining the pore. Changes in pH, therefore, can directly affect these proteins and their function.[38]

Although it is generally believed that water enters the red cell through a channel, there is disagreement as to which membrane protein(s) form this pore. Solomon et al[40] initially reported that tetramers of band 3 formed a channel through which water, chloride and nonelectrolytes moved. Band 3 is a 93-kD glycoprotein that appears as a diffuse band on SDS-PAGE. It exhibits great heterogeneity in its glycosylation which has been attributed to ABH and I activities.[41,42] Further digestion of its cytoplasmic portion using chymotrypsin or pronase, yields additional variation[43,44] indicating that another, yet undefined, genetic polymorphism may be present. Yu and Steck[45] postulated that band 3 may represent a class of related transmembrane proteins encompassing many transport functions. Some of the functions already attributed to band 3 are: anion transport, membrane binding of glyceraldehyde 3-P dehydrogenase, aldolase and hemoglobin, as well as being the attachment site for spectrin.

Macy [46] and Benga et al [47] suggested that band 4.5 might function as the urea transporter. Kasahara and Hinkle [48] have already implicated band 4.5 in glucose movement; they isolated and purified the D-glucose transporter from erythrocytes. It is a 55-kD glycoprotein that contains 5% neutral sugars, 7% glucosamine and 5% sialic acid which shows some heterogeneity. Whitfield et al [49] have suggested that this region contains four families of proteins, two of which have no known function.

The defect in the Jk(a−b−) red cells causing them to resist lysis in aqueous urea could either be due to urea or water movement, since both are involved in the urea lysis of red cells. Although Heaton et al [30] postulated that the defect was in urea transport, they gave no evidence to support this theory. The suggestion remained dormant for several years but the topic is now becoming of interest to membrane transport researchers. Edwards-Moulds and Kasschau [50] found that normal red cells treated with 1mM phloretin, an inhibitor of urea and glucose transport, had only 88.2% ± 10% lysis in 2M urea. When the same donors' cells were pretreated with p-chloromercuribenzene sulfonate (PCMBS), an inhibitor of urea and water movement, and incubated in 2M urea, hemolysis was reduced to 3.8% ± 2.4%. McGregor and McDougall [51] also used urea and water transport inhibitors and concluded that the defect in Jk:−3 red cells involved urea transport.

The results of urea transport studies are ambiguous. ^{14}C-labeled urea was used to study the urea uptake of normal and Jk(a−b−) red cells. [34,50] Urea appeared to move into the null erythrocytes, although the percent uptake of six different Jk(a−b−) donors was only 50-60% of normal. Other investigators, using thiourea and urea efflux studies, found the efflux rates of Jk(a−b−) red cells to be the same as normal cells in the presence of a competitive urea inhibitor, thionicotinamide. [52] They concluded that Jk(a−b−) red cells were devoid of mediated urea transport. Most recently, McDougall and McGregor [28] described a reverse urea lysis test. They preincubated Jk:−3 red cells in 2M urea/ 0.8% PBS for 5 minutes then decreased the extracellular urea concentration to 0.2M. This caused the Jk:−3 but not normal red cells to lyse. One should note that these reports are not all measuring the same parameters.

The question of abnormal urea versus water movement in the Jk(a−b−) red cells may need additional research before a full answer is found. Several observations cannot be fully explained by postulating the absence of the urea transporter in the null cells. The first is that at 300mM concentrations of urea prepared in water the average percent hemolysis of four Jk(a−b−) donor samples was 34.7%.[30] At concentrations ranging from 0.5M-10M there was no lysis using the same donor samples. Similar results were obtained using the reverse urea lysis test described by McDougall and McGregor[28] (Moulds J, unpublished observation). These results suggest that water movement across the membrane of Jk(a−b−) red cells may be restricted in the presence of urea and that only a small amount of urea is needed for this inhibition.

One may argue that red cells without a functional transporter would shrink and that the delay in lysis is the time it takes for urea to penetrate the lipid bilayer and cause osmotic lysis. Indeed, Heaton and McLoughlin[26] reported that the Jk(a−b−) cells they studied shrank and crenated in 2M urea. Others have not been able to duplicate these results using both light microscopy and phase-contrast video-imaging (O'Neill R, personal communication). By scanning electron microscopy the Jk(a−b−) erythrocytes appear swollen and spherocytic in 2M urea (Fig 4-5). This "rounding up" causes a decrease in red cell diameter.

Further studies with the Jk(a−b−) red cells may play a key role in the study of membrane transport systems. Toon and Solomon[53] have suggested that urea permeates the membrane through band 3 while water enters through another pathway, possibly band 4.5. More recently they[54] have postulated that bands 3 and 4.5 might form a complex through which urea, water and anions move. If this is the case, then an abnormal urea transport protein could also affect water transport. However, Fröhlich et al[55] have found chloride transport unaffected in Jk(a−b−) red cells, suggesting that band 3 of these cells is normal. Jk(a−b−) red cells should be instrumental in settling the arguments of urea/water movement and the responsible proteins. In addition, we may soon link another blood group antigen to a specific membrane protein and its function.

Genetic Models

The finding of the Jk(a−b−) phenotype was most easily explained by a third allele Jk which did not produce Kidd antigens.[18] Based on serological data and family studies, Issitt[56 (p 308-15)] suggested a simple model for the genetic control of the Kidd blood group antigens. The genes Jk^a, Jk^b and Jk would act on a precursor substance to produce Jk^a/Jk3, Jk^b/

THE KIDD BLOOD GROUP SYSTEM   85

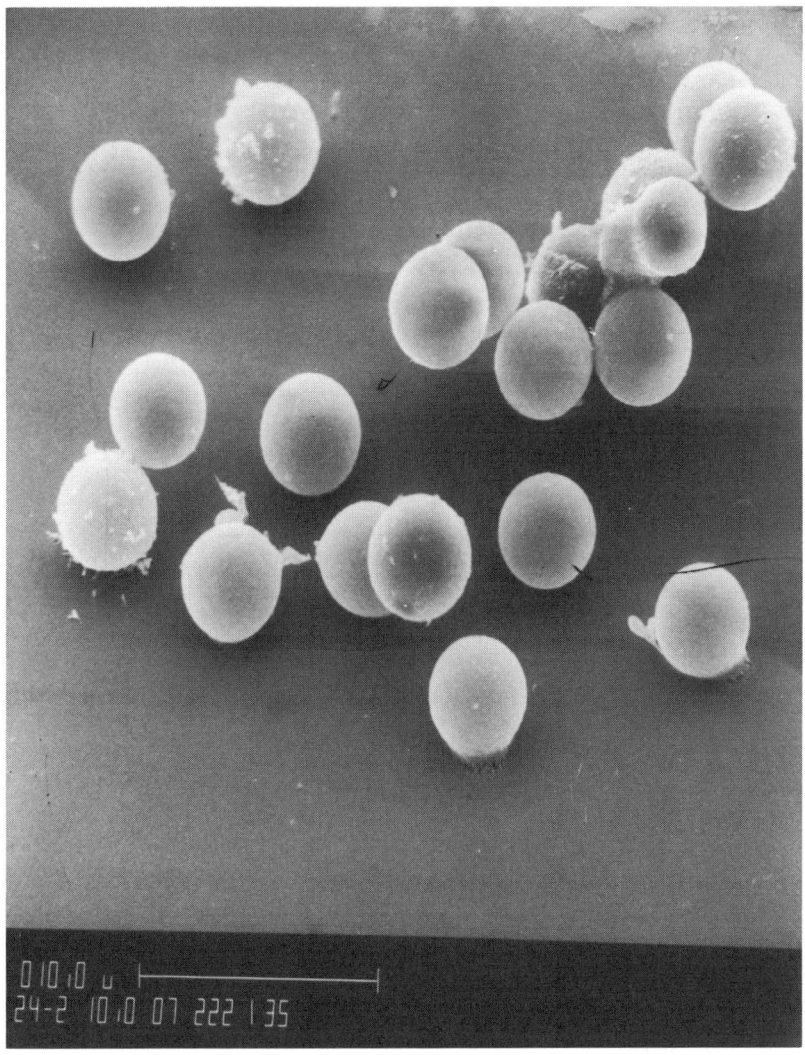

Figure 4-5. Scanning electron micrograph of Jk(a−b−) red cells incubated in 2M aqueous urea for 10 minutes. Magnification equals 2400x.

Jk and no antigens, respectively. More recently a suppressor gene, *In(Jk)*, has been described.[16]

The biochemical data do not entirely support the idea of Jk being a silent allele coding for no gene product. Of the numerous investigators who have run SDS-PAGE on membranes from various Jk(a−b−) donors, none have noted any deleted protein bands. If the urea transporter is band 3 or 4.5, as suggested, such a loss would certainly be noticed because it would adversely affect anion or glucose transport.

An alternative theory may be that *Jk* codes for a mutant protein containing an amino acid substitution resulting in a net charge difference. SDS-PAGE, which separates proteins by molecular weight, would not be able to detect such a change. PAGE without detergents will separate proteins based on weight and charge. It is interesting to note that Okubo et al[16] detected an additional 67-kD band using PAGE without SDS for both the *In(Jk)* and *JkJk* types. A change in the amino acid backbone of the Kidd glycoprotein might also affect its reactivity with anti-Jk^a and anti-Jk^b, thus these cells would appear to lack Kidd antigens.

How might this mutant protein affect urea and or water transport? The permeation of urea is thought to be highly dependent on H^+ bonding at the channel entrance.[33] Urea may bind in such a way with the abnormal protein that it causes a conformational change in the protein which hinders urea transport or closes water channels or both. Dorogi and Solomon[57] have already shown that urea can bind to band 3 causing a conformational change in that protein. In a similar manner, the sulfonylurea drugs depicted in Fig 4-1 may also bind to the membrane proteins carrying the Kidd antigens resulting in a conformational change and the appearance of "apparent auto-anti-Jk^a."

Disease Association

Some of the red cell blood group null phenotypes have been linked to hematological disorders and HLA has been multiply associated with numerous diseases. The Rh$_{null}$ individual reported by Schmidt and Vos[58] had a compensated hemolytic state. These red cells exhibited excessive lysis in osmotic fragility and auto-hemolysis tests. The McLeod phenotype was first associated with a disease state when it was found that some boys with chronic granulomatous disease also had this rare phenotype. Continued research has shown that some of these persons have a compensated hemolytic state[59] and that there is an association between the McLeod phenotype and Duchenne muscular dystrophy.[60]

The lack of association of the Jk(a−b−) phenotype with any particular disease may simply indicate that we have not looked in the right direction. The most persuasive evidence for normality in this rare phenotype are the blood donors themselves. None of the 66 Polynesian Jk (a−b−) donors[20] or the 14 Japanese[16] exhibited any abnormalities that could be detected by routine donor screening. In addition, many of the reported cases of anti-Jk3 have been found during pregnancy, which can hardly be considered a disease state.

Moulds[24] performed hematological tests on four Jk(a−b−) donors. Tests included: red cell count, white cell count, hemoglobin, hematocrit, red cell indices, platelet count, reticulocyte count, plasma haptoglobin levels, direct antiglobulin test, differential and scanning electron microscopy (SEM) of blood smears, and osmotic fragilities (immediate and after 24-hr incubation at 37 C). Results from each donor were within normal ranges except for one male who exhibited decreased hemoglobin/hematocrit, decreased mean corpuscular volume and mean corpuscular hemoglobin content as well as slightly elevated red cell distribution width and reticulocyte count. These results, along with the decreased osmotic fragility, were consistent with a previous diagnosis of β-thalassemia minor.

In addition, one female showed some stomatocytes on SEM. Although the same results were obtained on a fresh sample this morphology was not evident by Wright's stain. With the exception of the donor with thalassemia trait, none of the Jk(a−b−) donors studied displayed any gross hematological abnormalities nor evidence of accelerated red cell destruction. In a study of three other Jk(a−b−) donors at the New York Blood Center, there was no indication of increased in vivo cell destruction.[15]

It is hard to believe that cells having abnormal urea transport would not exhibit some pathological findings, but to date there is no such evidence. Although the specialized transport of urea does not appear to fulfill any significant physiological function in the human red cell, Macey[46] has postulated that rapid transport of urea may be necessary in the renal circulation. Circulating red cells are exposed to high concentrations of urea and sodium in the renal medulla. A red cell with poor urea transport would be in danger of hypertonic lysis. Upon emerging, the urea-loaded cell could be faced with the opposite problem. Therefore, the role of urea transport in the red cell may be to preserve the cell's osmotic stability and membrane deformability.

If movement of urea and water is mediated through band 3 as Solomon has postulated, kidney cells may also be suspect since band 3 has been found in the rat kidney.[61] Two Jk(a−b−) donors tested to date have had normal serum electrolytes, blood urea nitrogen and creatinine (Moulds J, unpublished observations) but further tests of kidney function are in progress. Maybe from these we will gain a better idea of the exact function of the Kidd antigens and their role in health and disease.

Conclusion

The Kidd blood group system, dormant for so long, is now coming to life. Resistance to urea lysis found with Jk(a−b−) red cells is under further study by membrane biologists. Molecular geneticists are attempting to clone the Kidd genes while physicians search for disease associations. We can certainly expect some interesting information to appear in the next few years for what once seemed another mundane blood group.

References

1. Sosler SD, Behzad O, Garratty G, Lee CL, Postoway N, Khomo O. Acute hemolytic anemia associated with a chlorpropamide-induced apparent auto-anti-Jk^a. Transfusion 1984;24:206-9.
2. Logue GL, Boyd AE, Rosse WF. Chlorpropamide-induced immune hemolytic anemia. N Engl J Med 1970;283:900-4.
3. Bird GWG, Eeles GH, Litchfield JA, Rahman M, Wingham J. Haemolytic anaemia associated with antibodies to tolbutamide. Br Med J 1972;1:728-9.
4. Garratty G. Problems in pretransfusion tests related to drugs and chemical. Am J Med Tech 1976;42:209-19.
5. Halima D, Garratty G, Bueno R. An apparent anti-Jk^a reacting only in the presence of methyl esters of hydroxybenzoic acid. Transfusion 1982;22:521-4.
6. Judd WJ, Steiner EA, Cochran RK. Paraben-associated autoanti-Jk^a antibodies. Three examples detected using commercially prepared low-ionic-strength saline containing parabens. Transfusion 1982;22:31-5.
7. Masouredis SP, Sudora E, Mahan L, Victoria EJ. Quantitative immunoferritin microscopy of Fy^a, Fy^b, Jk^a, U and Di^b antigen site numbers in human red cells. Blood 1980;56:969-77.
8. Marsh WL, Øyen R, Nichols ME. Kidd blood-group antigens of leukocytes and platelets. Transfusion 1974;14:378-81.
9. Gaidulis L, Branch DR, Lazar GS, Petz LD, Blume KG. The red cell antigens A, B, D, U, Gerbich (Ge), Jk^{a}Jk^b

(Jk3), and Cartwright (Yt[a]) are not detected on human granulocytes. Br J Haematol 1985;60:659-68.
10. Dunstan RA, Simpson MB, Rosse WF. Erythrocyte antigens on human platelets. Absence of Rh, Duffy, Kell, Kidd, and Lutheran antigens. Transfusion 1984;24: 243-6.
11. Dunstan RA. Status of major red cell blood group antigens on neutrophils, lymphocytes, and monocytes. Br J Haematol 1986;62:301-9.
12. Habibi B, Avril J, Fouillade MT, Lopez M, Vaucelle R, Salmon C. Jk(a−b−) phenotype in a French family. Quantitative evidence for the inheritance of a silent allele (Jk). Haematologia 1976;10:403-10.
13. McGinnis MH, Leiberman R, Holland PV. The Jk[b] red cell antigen and gram negative organisms (abstract). Transfusion 1979;19:663.
14. McGinnis MH. The ubiquitous nature of human blood group antigens as evidenced by bacterial, viral and parasitic infections. In: Garratty G, ed. Blood group antigens and disease. Arlington, VA: American Association of Blood Banks, 1983:25-43.
15. Marsh WL. Deleted antigens of the Rhesus and Kell blood groups: association with cell membrane defects. In: Garratty G, ed. Blood group antigens and disease. Arlington, VA: American Association of Blood Banks, 1983;165-85.
16. Okubo Y, Yamaguchi H, Nagao N, Tomita T, Seno T, Tanaka M. Heterogeneity of the phenotype Jk(a−b−) found in Japanese. Transfusion 1986;26:237-9.
17. Sinor LT, Eastwood KL, Plapp FV. Dot-blot purification of the Kidd blood group antigen. Med Lab Sci 1987;44: 294-6.
18. Pinkerton FJ, Mermod LE, Liles BA, Jack JA Jr, Noudes J. The phenotype Jk(a−b−) in the Kidd blood group system. Vox Sang 1959;4:155-60.
19. Crawford MN, Greenwalt TJ, Sasaki T, Tippet P, Sanger R, Race RR. The phenotype Lu(a−b−) together with unconventional Kidd groups in one family. Transfusion 1961;1:228-32.
20. Woodfield DG, Douglas R, Smith J, Simpson A, Pinder L, Staveley JM. The Jk(a−b−) phenotype in New Zealand Polynesians. Transfusion 1982;22:276-8.
21. Mizui M, Uchiyama E, Kikuchi M, et al. First example of the rare blood phenotype Jk(a−b−) and incidence of the phenotype in Japanese population (abstract). Jpn J Hum Genet 1983;28:118.

22. Klarkowski DB. An avid anti-Jk3 antibody detected in a Jk(a−b−) Caucasian propositus: an unusual prenatal finding. Aust J Med Lab Sci 1984;5:26-7.
23. Sistonen P. The Jk(a−b−) phenotype in a Finnish family. Abstracts of the 18th Congress of the International Society of Blood Transfusion. Munich, West Germany: 1984:164.
24. Moulds J. The role of the Kidd blood group antigens in red cell membrane permeability. (Thesis) Houston, TX: University of Houston at Clear Lake, 1986.
25. Obarski G, Hartnett PL, Prewitt PL, Issitt PD. The Jk(a−b−) phenotype, probably occurring as a transient phenomenon (abstract). Transfusion 1987;27:548.
26. Heaton DC, McLoughlin K. Jk(a−b−) red blood cells resist urea lysis. Transfusion 1982;22:70-1.
27. Lyne CJ. Jk(a−b−): blood group gems of the South Pacific. N Zea J Med Lab Tech 1985;39:115-6.
28. McDougall DCJ, McGregor M. Jk:−3 red cells have a defect in urea transport: a new urea-dependent lysis test. Transfusion 1988;28:197-8.
29. Edwards-Moulds J, Kasschau M. The effect of lytic agents on Jk(a−b−) red cells. Abstracts of the 21st Congress of the International Society of Haematology and 19th Congress of the International Society Blood Transfusion. Sydney, Australia: 1986:357.
30. Heaton DC, Wong LT, McLoughlin K. The Jk(a−b−) phenotype and urea transport. Abstracts of the 19th Congress of the International Society of Haematology and 17th Congress of the International Society of Blood Transfusion. Budapest, Hungary: 1982:222.
31. Maynard RR, Levitt DG. Red cell membrane transport systems. J Gen Physiol 1983;81:228-37.
32. Jay AWL, Rowlands S. The stages of osmotic haemolysis. J Physiol 1975;252:817-32.
33. Sha'afi RI, Gary-Bobo CM, Solomon AK. Permeability of red cell membranes to small hydrophobic and lipophilic solutes. J Gen Physiol 1971;58:238-58.
34. Edwards-Moulds J, Kasschau M. A mechanism by which Jk(a−b−) red cells resist lysis in 2M urea. Transfusion 1986;26:561.
35. Edwards-Moulds J, Kasschau M. Methods for the detection of *Jk* heterozygotes: interpretations and applications. Transfusion (in press).
36. Macey RI. Transport of water and nonelectrolytes across red cell membranes. In: Tosteson DC, ed. Membrane

transport in biology. II. Transport across single biological membranes. Berlin: Springer-Verlag, 1979:1-57.
37. Solomon AK. Characterization of biological membranes by equivalent pores. J Gen Physiol 1968;51:335S.
38. Nathan DG, Shohet SB. Erythrocyte ion transport defects and hemolytic anemia: "hydrocytosis" and "desiccytosis." Semin Hematol 1970;7:381-408.
39. Sha'afi RI. Water and small nonelectrolyte permeation in red cells. In: Ellory JL, Lew V, eds. Membrane transport in red cells. London: Academic Press, 1977:221-56.
40. Solomon AK, Chasan B, Dix JA, et al. The aqueous pore in the red cell membrane: band 3 as a channel for anions, cations, nonelectrolytes and water. In: Kummerow FA, Benga G, Holmes RP, eds. Biomembranes and cell functions, vol 414. New York: Annals of the New York Academy of Science, 1983:93-124.
41. Tanner MTA, Boxer DH. Separation and some properties of the major protein of the human erythrocyte membrane. Biochem J 1972;129:333-47.
42. Tsuji T, Irimura T, Osawa T. The carbohydrate moiety of band-3 glycoprotein of the human erythrocyte membrane. Biochem J 1980;187:677-86.
43. Singh MK, Kahler H, Steck TL. Primary structural analysis of a 23,000 dalton fragment of band 3, a protein of the human red cell membrane (abstract). Fed Proc 1978;37:1507.
44. Mueller TJ, Morrison M. Detection of a variant protein 3, the major transmembrane protein of the human erythrocyte. J Biol Chem 1977;252:6573-6.
45. Yu J, Steck TL. Isolation and characterization of band 3, the predominant polypeptide of the human erythrocyte membrane. J Biol Chem 1975;250:9170-5.
46. Macey RI. Transport of urea and water in red blood cells. Am J physiol 1984;246:C195-203.
47. Benga G, Pop VI, Popescu O, Ionescu M, Mihele V. Water exchange through erythrocyte membranes: nuclear magnetic resonance studies on the effects of inhibitors and of chemical modification of human membranes. J Membr Biol 1983;76:129-37.
48. Kasahara M, Hinkle PC. Reconstitution and purification of the D-glucose transporter from human erythrocytes. J Biol Chem 1977;252:7384-90.
49. Whitfield CF, Coleman DB, Kay MMB, Shiffer KA, Goodman SR. Human erythrocyte membrane proteins of zone 4.5 exist as families of related proteins. Am J Physiol 1985;248:C70-9.

50. Edwards-Moulds J, Kasschau M. The effect of 2 molar urea on Jk(a–b–) red cells. Vox Sang 1988 (in press).
51. McGregor M, McDougall DCJ. Investigations of the movement of urea across the red cell membrane of normal and Jk:–3 cells. Abstracts of the British Blood Transfusion Society. Stirling, England: 1987.
52. Fröhlich O, Gunn RB, Gargus JJ, Rizzolo LJ. Urea and thiourea transport in normal and Jk(a–b–) erythrocytes. Biophys J 1988;53:531A.
53. Toon MR, Solomon AK. Control of red cell urea and water permeability by sulfhydryl groups. Biochem Biophys Acta 1986;860:361-75.
54. Toon MR, Solomon AK. Modulation of water and urea transport in red cells: effects of pH and phloretin. J Membr Biol 1987;99:157-64.
55. Fröhlich O, Jones SC. Denaturation of a membrane transport protein by urea: the erythrocyte anion exchanger. J Membr Biol 1987;98:33-42.
56. Issitt PD. Blood group serology, 3rd ed. Miami: Montgomery Scientific, 1985.
57. Dorogi PL, Solomon AK. Interactions of thiourea with band 3 in human red cell membranes. J Membr Biol 1985;85:37-48.
58. Schmidt PJ, Vos GH. Multiple phenotype abnormalities associated with Rh null (– – –/– – –). Vox Sang 1967;13:18-20.
59. Wimer BM, Marsh WL, Taswell HF, et al. Hematological changes associated with the McLeod phenotype of the Kell blood group system. Br J Haematol 1977;36:219-24.
60. Marsh WL, Marsh NJ, Moore A, et al. Elevated serum creatinine phosphokinase in subjects with McLeod syndrome. Vox Sang 1981;40:403-11.
61. Drenckham D, Schulter K, Allen D, Bennett V. Colocalization of band 3 with ankyrin and spectrin at the basal membrane of intercalated cells in the rat kidney. Science 1985;230:1287-9.

In: Pierce, SR, and Macpherson, CR, eds.
Blood Group Systems: Duffy, Kidd and Lutheran
Arlington, VA: American Association
of Blood Banks, 1988

5

The Lutheran Blood Group System: Serology and Genetics

Mary N. Crawford, MD

IN ENGLAND, IN 1945, an extraordinary patient was found to have five antibodies, three of which were new to the blood banking world. Besides anti-c and anti-N, the investigators found the first example of anti-C^w, another antibody they called anti-Levay (which 33 years later was recognized as the first case of anti-Kp^c) and the new Lutheran antibody. The name "Lutheran" honored the implicated donor of the cells that reacted with this antibody in the multiply transfused patient.

The rapid addition of new blood groups during that era created a dearth of letters by which to identify them, so an agreement was reached to use two letters plus the superscripts "a" and "b." This first member of the Lutheran system was, therefore, called Lu^a. The anticipated allele was to be termed Lu^b.[1] Ten years passed before patients were found with antibodies fitting the allelic pattern for anti-Lu^b.[2]

The system remained comfortably contained as a two-allele concept until 1959 when a family was found with several members who lacked both Lu^a and Lu^b on their red cells. Studies of two generations strongly suggested that a dominant suppressor was responsible for the null phenotype. This was a peculiarity previously unknown for blood groups.[3]

Within two years another null phenotype was found in a patient with tuberculosis. Her antibody was reactive with all cells except those of the family with the suppressed Lutheran type. No compatible cells could be found for the patient among her relatives. This null phenotype appeared to be genetically recessive.[4]

During the next few years a number of high frequency antibodies were seen which were negative only with Lu(a−b−)

Mary N. Crawford, MD, Pearson C. Cummin Memorial Laboratory, Villanova, Pennsylvania cells, but which were reactive with each other. A variety of Lutheran-related antibodies were identified, leading to a nomenclature of numbers.[5] Over the ensuing years the list has grown to almost 20. And two new sets of alleles have emerged within the Lutheran system. The high frequency antigen Lu:6 was matched with the low frequency antigen Lu:9, and Lu:8 was paired with Lu:14.[6,7]

Linkage of two inherited characters and "crossing-over" between them were first demonstrated with the Lutheran system. Several decades passed before the system could be assigned to chromosome 19.[8,9]

Common Lutheran Phenotypes and Frequencies

Lu^a

The patient who initiated the Lutheran system, and whose antibody eventually was designated anti-Lu^a was a 25-year-old female who had never been pregnant. Her disease, lupus erythematosus diffusus, led to a persistent anemia for which she received nine units of blood over an extended period. The Lutheran antibody appeared after the third transfusion and the cells of the donor of the third unit reacted with the new antibody. Screening of random English donors revealed a frequency of about 8% for the Lutheran antigen. Family studies indicated it was inherited as a dominant factor and that Lutheran was not linked to ABO, Rh, MN or P. Later studies also excluded linkage with the Kell and Lewis blood groups.

The anti-Lu^a gradually weakened and had almost disappeared within 2 months. An attempt to immunize one donor to this Lutheran antigen failed to create the antibody. During the next year, the original patient was injected with small amounts of blood from an Lu(a+) donor in hopes of reviving the antibody. Six injections were ineffective. Five weeks later seven more injections were given, which produced a potent anti-N.[10]

Eventually, eight more Lu(a−) patients, without a history of blood group antibodies, were selected for transfusion with Lu(a+) blood. Each patient received one or two units without any adverse reactions. Their sera were tested every 2 weeks for 2 months. Two patients produced anti-Lu^a and no other antibodies were detected. These two patients had been previously transfused but, in one case, all the earlier donors were recalled and found to be Lu(a−). The antibodies lasted only a short time in these patients. The weaker one was gone in

44 days and the titer of the other, 2 weeks after transfusion, was 16; it dropped to 2 in another 2 weeks.[11]

In 1948, a second example of anti-Lu^a was reported in a 38-year-old patient with cirrhosis whose serum also demonstrated anti-D. The anti-Lu^a had a titer of 16 although all recent donors were found to be Lu(a−). The patient was given small amounts of Lu(a+) cells over a 2 month period but the crossmatches were compatible with these cells. One year later the titer was 1. The antibody was undetectable after another year. The third example of anti-Lu^a, which appeared to be naturally occurring was reported in 1950.[12]

Testing large numbers of random Caucasian populations has produced a frequency of 7-8% for the Lu^a antigen, except in a Mennonite population which had a frequency of about 14%.[13] In a study of 991 random American Black donors, 52 were Lu(a+) for a frequency of 5.2% (author's laboratory). The Lu^a antigen has not yet been reported in Asians, Eskimos or Australian aborigines.[1]

Three examples of anti-Lu^a were found in 18,613 random donors in Milwaukee. These appeared to be naturally occurring antibodies.[14]

Lu^b

The long anticipated antibody for Lu^b was reported in 1956 with the title "The expected blood-group antibody, anti-Lu^b."[2] The patient had had three normal pregnancies and no transfusions. Her cells were Lu(a+) and her antibody titers were weaker with cells that reacted with both anti-Lu^a and her antibody.

The second example of anti-Lu^b was reported soon after the first. The patient was a 27-year-old woman who had had three normal pregnancies but was given one unit of blood for anemia 2 weeks before the birth of the third child. A second blood unit was given 16 months later. After another 3 years the patient had vaginal bleeding with miscarriage of the fourth pregnancy. Four units of blood were transfused with a rise in hemoglobin from 8.5 g/dl to 11.0 g/dl. A week later the patient became jaundiced. After a few days the icterus faded and the hemoglobin, which had fallen to 8.8 g/dl, spontaneously rose to 14.8 g/dl over the next 5 weeks. The patient's serum strongly agglutinated all panel cells at 37 C and with antihuman globulin (AHG). At the time this case was published the patient's parents were thought to exhibit the rare mating of Lu(a+b+)

and Lu(a+b−), but when retested in later years with stronger sera, both were found to be Lu(a+b+). The patient and all three siblings (identical twins included) typed as Lu(a+b−). The patient's antibody was negative with the cells of the first patient with anti-Lu^b and with those of her ABO-compatible sibling. The serum was also negative with cells from two of the children from an Lu(a+) by Lu(a+) mating studied in earlier years with anti-Lu^a sera.[14]

In 1967, a review of the Lutheran blood groups included a list of 12 anti-Lu^a sera and 32 anti-Lu^b sera.[15] The paper also included many titrations in an unsuccessful search for the silent Lutheran allele. The review contains useful data on the development of Lutheran antigen expression on red cells, the obstetrical and transfusion histories of the antibody producers, the clinical effects in patients and newborns and the serological characteristics of the antibodies. In the collection of patients with anti-Lu^a, nine of the 12 were male and four had never been transfused. Of those with anti-Lu^b, 28 of the 32 were female. All four males had been transfused; 13 of the women had been transfused and at least nine of these had also had one or more pregnancies. Ten of the women had never been transfused and had been immunized by one or more pregnancies. Five had incomplete histories, but four of them had been pregnant.[15]

The extensive British and European studies with anti-Lu^a indicated that the Lu(a+b−) phenotype would have a frequency of 0.15%. This figure has remained valid.[1]

Lutheran Null Phenotypes

In(Lu): Dominant Suppressor

The tidy Lutheran system was jolted in 1959 by a red cell specimen that was negative with anti-Lu^a and anti-Lu^b sera. Because the cells belonged to a healthy investigator in the blood grouping field, family studies were expedited. Both siblings and the father were also negative for Lu^a and Lu^b, as were two first cousins. A niece carried the null phenotype into the third generation. It was soon apparent that a dominant gene was suppressing expression of the Lutheran antigens.[3] In ensuing years the family (Cr.) has grown into the fourth generation and now lists 10 Lu(a−b−) members. Over the years a number of similar families have been studied. This form of null phenotype was unknown in other blood groups.

Studies on the Cr. family and all similar kindred disclosed that the Lu(a−b−) members were almost always negative with the only known example of anti-Auberger (Au^a), although only 20% of Caucasians should be. The Lutheran-positive members of these families fell within the usual Auberger percentages.[16] This has proved true with a more recent example of anti-Au^a. Early tests of the Cr. family had also led to some disagreement about P$_1$ typings and a comment that the proposita possessed a normal "grown-up" I antigen but had an exceedingly weak i antigen. Nothing more was done about these findings until 1973 when a burst of activity demonstrated that persons with dominant suppression of their Lutheran types were almost always suppressed for P$_1$, i and Au^a. Such suppression was not found with the recessive form of Lu$_{null}$ (see below).[17]

Proof that Lu^a was also suppressed had to await a family with the Lu^a gene. Studies on two families showing suppression of Lu^a were reported in 1971 and 1973.[18, 19] In one of these families it was clearly shown that the suppressor gene was not part of the Lutheran locus. The term In(Lu) was introduced to distinguish the "inhibited" form of Lu(a−b−) from the recessive form.[19]

LuLu: Recessive Lu$_{Null}$

In 1961, the serum of an English patient (L. B.), who had received one unit of blood 11 years earlier for a lobectomy and now was due for a thoracoplasty, was found to be incompatible with all red cells except those of the Cr. family. The patient's cells were then found to be Lu(a−b−). Her two children and one living parent were Lu(a−b+); and no other relatives had the null phenotype. However, dosage studies with the children's cells suggested they had inherited a single Lu^b antigen and that L. B. had, therefore, a recessive form of Lu$_{null}$. The patient's antibody was active at room temperature and 37 C and reactive by saline, albumin and AHG techniques. Her antibody behaved as an inseparable anti-Lu^{a}Lu^b, which in later years was dubbed anti-Lu3. L. B. underwent successful surgery during which she received a unit of her own blood and one unit from the Cr. family. She received much publicity but had no adverse reactions.[4]

Later investigators demonstrated that, with suitable Lutheran antibodies, the red cells of most persons with the Lu(a−b−) phenotype of the suppressed form would adsorb and elute anti-Lu^b and anti-Lu^a, if the genes for these antigens were present.[20] In another study, the red cells of two related individuals with the recessive form of Lu(a−b−) would not adsorb and elute Lutheran antibodies.[18]

L. B.'s serum was used to screen over 18,000 random donors. One Lu(a−b−) donor (S.H.) was found. S.H. had no antibodies. Her father and one of her two siblings were also Lu(a−b−), indicating that the family was exhibiting the "suppressed" form of Lu_{null}.[4]

Several years passed before any other examples of the recessive form were found. Then a very large inbred Caucasian kindred from Nova Scotia produced three Lu(a−b−) members, two females and one male. The two females had made anti-$Lu^a Lu^b$ (Lu3).[21] The same antibody and null phenotype were also found in one American Black woman (H.H.) and in a Japanese man (H.F.). Very few of the relatives in the family of H.H. could be tested and no Lu(a−b−) members were found. The family of H.F. (32 members in all) was extensively tested, and only his sister demonstrated the Lu(a−b−) type. Their parents were first cousins once removed, and the kindred could be traced for six generations.[1, 22]

These studies confirmed a recessive type of Lu_{null}.[1] This Lu_{null} phenotype was not passed on to each generation as was the *In(Lu)* type. The presence of an *LuLu* genotype was shown by the failure of those persons to pass on either Lu^a or Lu^b, as would be expected in the *In(Lu)* type.

Adsorption and elution testing has shown that *In(Lu)* individuals possess small amounts of the Lutheran antigens, and family studies have demonstrated transmission of functional *Lutheran* genes to offspring who have not inherited the independent *In(Lu)* suppressor gene. Therefore it seems unlikely that those with the In(Lu) phenotype can make anti-Lu3 or any of the Lutheran-related high frequency antibodies (see below).[18, 19, 23]

X-Linked Lu_{null}

The Lu_{null} classifications remained essentially unchanged until an exciting report appeared in 1986 describing a third genetic form of the Lu(a−b−) phenotype which was shown to be X-borne.[24] A White Australian male was singled out of a mass screening for rare blood donors because he was Wr(a+). He was then also found to be Lu(a−b−), so his family was studied. One member of the first generation was available for testing and many members of the second and third generations, 50 in all, were studied.

The red cells of the propositus resembled those of *In(Lu)* individuals in several ways. They adsorbed and eluted anti-Lu^b and were Au(a−) and weak for P_1; and there were no

Table 5-1. Suppressed, Recessive and X-Borne Lu$_{null}$ Differences

	In(Lu)	Recessive	X-Borne
Adsorption and elution of Lu antibodies from cells	yes	no	yes
Production of antibodies	no	yes	no
Lu(a−b−) phenotype in family members	*	sibs.†	‡
Depression of Au^a and P$_1$	most	no§	§
Expression of i	depressed	normal	enhanced
Reactions with monoclonal antibodies (eg, H86, M447)	no	yes	yes

*The Lu(a−b−) phenotype will be found in one parent and probably also in some siblings and offspring.
†The Lu(a−b−) phenotype, unless there is consanguinity, will be found only, if at all, in siblings.
‡The Lu(a−b−) type will not be found in parents, but may be found in brothers and sons of sisters.
§Insufficient examples for study.

atypical antibodies in the six Lu(a−b−) members in generations II and III. However, they differed from *In(Lu)* cells in having enhanced i and depressed I antigen expression and in being reactive with the monoclonal antibodies H86 and M447, and with anti-Wj (see Chapter 6). All six Lu(a−b−) family members were male.

The inheritance was unusual in that three Lu(a−b−) members, two siblings and one first cousin, had mothers and fathers who were Lu(a−b+), thereby differing from the *In(Lu)* form of inheritance. The amorphic recessive form of inheritance could be eliminated because five unrelated persons would have had to carry the very rare amorphic gene in a family with no history of consanguinity. An X-borne recessive inhibitor of the products of the Lutheran locus seemed likely. The term *XS* was suggested for the locus on the X chromosome, *XS1* to represent the common allele permitting Lutheran expression, and *XS2* for the rare allele inhibiting expression of the Lutheran antigens.[24] The three forms of Lu$_{null}$ are categorized in Table 5-1.

Frequency of Lu$_{null}$

Because only one Lu(a−b−) sample was found when 18,000 random donors were screened with L.B.'s serum in Sheffield, England, the possessors of this type could consider themselves truly unusual. In later years the *In(Lu)* individuals lost some of their distinction. Using anti-Lu^b, 250,000 random donors were tested in England. About one in 3000 was found to be negative with both anti-Lu^a and anti-Lu^b.[25] Another study was carried out in Houston, Texas using a monoclonal antibody. In this donor population of 42,000 there were eight Lu(a−b−) cells. The Houston cohort (donors and relatives) exhibited varying degrees of serological and membrane defects.[26]

The recessive form of Lu(a−b−) is indeed rare. Most of these individuals will be recognized only after production of anti-Lu3 following pregnancy or transfusion. Only one family has been reported with the X-borne Lu(a−b−) phenotype. It must be exceedingly rare.

High Frequency Lutheran-Related Antigens and Their Antibodies

Increasing complexity for the system has been marked by the steady addition of new antibodies to high frequency antigens that appear related to Lutheran. The term "para-Lutheran" was applied to this collection to avoid a genetic connotation since there was no proof of control by the *Lutheran* locus. The first of these to be published was given the label of anti-Lu4 and numerical nomenclature then became the rule for expansion of the blood group.[27]

The patient was Caucasian. She had had two pregnancies and had been transfused. Her antibody reacted with all except the dominant and recessive Lu(a−b−) red cells and those of two of her five siblings. She and her compatible siblings were Lu(a−b+). Red cells from her two children had normal titration scores with anti-Lu^b. Her parents were dead and there was no history of consanguinity. Reactions with cord cells were weaker than those of adult cells with the Lu4 antibody. Almost 3000 random blood donors were tested without finding compatible cells. An unsuccessful attempt was made to raise an allelic antibody by injecting two rabbits 10 times with Lu:−4 red cells.

By 1970 a number of laboratories had antibodies, from individuals with "normal" Lutheran phenotypes, which reacted with all except Lu(a−b−) red cells. At a "wet" workshop sponsored by the American Association of Blood Banks, investigators exchanged sera and cells. It was then possible to sort some of these antibodies into three new Lutheran classifications. The new antibodies became anti-Lu5, anti-Lu6 and anti-Lu7.[5] All three could be adsorbed and recovered from dominant Lu(a−b−) cells.

Two examples of anti-Lu5 were compatible with each other but reactive with all tested red cells except Lu(a−b−) of both dominant and recessive types. No compatible siblings were found. Both women had been pregnant and had been transfused. One was Black and the other White.

The anti-Lu6 was made by a Canadian woman of Polish birth. Two of her four siblings were Lu:−6. The patient and her compatible siblings had Lu^b antigens of normal strength.

The anti-Lu7 was made by a Caucasian woman who had never been transfused but had had five pregnancies. One of her three siblings was also Lu:−7.

In 1972 anti-Lu8 was reported in a Caucasian woman who had had three pregnancies and multiple transfusions. This antibody followed the patterns described above, being compatible only with both Lu$_{null}$ phenotypes and with two of her four siblings. Her parents and children were Lu:8. The proposita and her family were Lu(a−b+). The Lu:8 parents, siblings, two children and the daughter of one compatible sister reacted more weakly with anti-Lu8, suggesting heterozygosity.[28]

Anti-Lu11 was found in a 56-year-old Caucasian woman who had had four children and earlier transfusions without any problems or antibodies. While being treated for a lymphoma she was found to have a high frequency antibody that was reactive with all but Lu(a−b−) red cells of either dominant or recessive types. Her children and two siblings were incompatible as were all other red cells of high frequency, Lutheran-related phenotypes. She was given *In(Lu)* blood but died of her disease before the efficacy of the transfusion could be evaluated. The antibody appeared to be IgM and the agglutination resembled that of Lu^a in having some free cells (see below).[29]

The Lu12 number was reserved for Mrs. Much.'s antibody which reacted with all red cells except her own, one sister's and Lu$_{null}$ samples. Mrs. Much. was unusual, however, in being Lu(a−) but having a very weak Lu^b antigen. Her father and the compatible sister also had the Lu(a−b^w) phenotype.

Mrs. Much.'s serum reacted with red cells lacking the antigens Lu4, Lu5, Lu6, Lu7, Lu8 and Anton (see Chapter 6: "Anton" has been stripped of its Lu15 designation). The antibody reacted weakly with Mrs. Much.'s father's cells and with one Lu(a−b^w) cell sample found by screening 1050 donors in the province of Alberta.

Mrs. Much.'s Lu(a−b^w) red cells were weakly reactive with anti-Lu5, anti-Lu7, anti-Lu8, anti-Lu11 and anti-Lu13. The red cells of Mrs. Much., her father and her compatible sister failed to react with some examples of anti-Lu^b although the cells would adsorb and elute anti-Lu^b. Mrs. Much., her father and the compatible sister were P$_1$. The mother and the incompatible sister were P$_1$ negative. The family, of Polish and Ukrainian background, had no history of consanguinity.

Secretor studies of the family demonstrated segregation. Mrs. Much., her father and her incompatible brother were "secretors," whereas the compatible sister was a "non-secretor." The *Lutheran* genes were not segregating, therefore it was unlikely that the *Much.* gene was at the Lutheran locus.

Mrs. Much.'s first pregnancy had aborted at three months. She had never been transfused. Her antibody was found during her second pregnancy, which resulted in a healthy baby with no evidence of hemolytic disease of the newborn (HDN). The antibody reacted well with IgG AHG and by saline capillary tube tests.[30]

Lu13 is a number in quarantine. It is an unpublished antibody, made by a patient named Hughes; it reacts with all samples except the patient's own and Lu$_{null}$ red cells.[23] Several papers briefly mention it. Much.'s Lu:−12 cells reacted strongly with the Anton serum but weakly with anti-Lu13.[30] A patient with advanced Hodgkin's disease had a transient Wj− phenotype and anti-Wj in the serum. Although the patient and two siblings who typed as Wj+ were Lu:−13, there was no separable anti-Lu13 in the patient's serum.[23] (See Chapter 6.)

Anti-Lu16 was described in 1980. This antibody has been found in three Black females, all of whom typed as Lu(a+b−). The three are mutually compatible and negative with both dominant and recessive forms of Lu$_{null}$. Family studies could be carried out for only one of the cases and proved uninformative for linkage to Lutheran or any other system. In the family studied, both parents of the propositus and her four children were Lu(a+b+). There were no siblings. These cases were also unusual in that all three made anti-Lu^b as well as anti-Lu16.[23]

In 1979 another antibody reactive with all but Lu$_{null}$ cells was tagged as anti-Lu17.[31] Additional studies for this patient were reported in 1986 when her antibody was found to resemble those of the "high-titer, low-avidity" set in having weak agglutination to a titer of 256. For a red cell chromium survival test the patient was injected with Lu:17 cells, which had a shortened life span of 12.5 days.[32]

The incidence of these Lutheran antigens is unknown. Without mass screening of random populations or the discovery of lower frequency alleles for them, their frequency cannot be projected.

Allelic Lutheran Pairs

Interest in the Lutheran system increased with the discovery of two low frequency antigens allelic to two of the previously described high frequency antigens, which elevated them to true Lutheran status.

Lu6 and Lu9

It seemed pure luck that while the original Lu:−6 proposita (Mrs. Jank.) was undergoing further study a patient (Mrs. Mull), with anti-Lu^a and an unsolved antibody for a low frequency antigen, was also at hand. Mrs. Mull's serum strongly agglutinated Mrs. Jank.'s cells as well as the cells of the second Lu:−6 case (Mrs. Urs.). Blood samples were obtained from Poland from six of Mrs. Jank.'s siblings. Two of the siblings were Lu:−6 and reactive with Mrs. Mull's serum, three were positive with both sera and one was Lu:6 and negative with the Mull serum. All members were Lu(a−b+). Mrs. Mull's antibody was named anti-Lu9, that being the next available Lutheran number.[6]

The Mull family was extensively studied and proved to be very rewarding genetically. Three generations were available. Mr. Mull was Lu:9, as was his mother and the three Mull children. In the first generation, six of nine members were Lu:9. Two of Mr. Mull's five siblings were Lu:9 and 12 of 14 were Lu:9 in the third generation. The Lu:9 red cells of Mr. Mull's mother were found to be negative with 52 sera detecting low frequency antigens. Furthermore, the Mull family showed that Lu9, and therefore Lu6, were controlled by the Lutheran locus. Mr. Mull and his two Lu:9 siblings were Lu(a+b+).

The Mull pedigree (Fig 5-1) shows that the 14 children of the third generation were the result of three double backcross matings. Twelve children were Lu:9 but Lu(a−) and two children were Lu:−9 and Lu(a+). There were no recombinants and the lod score for the family was 6.3. Surprisingly, the

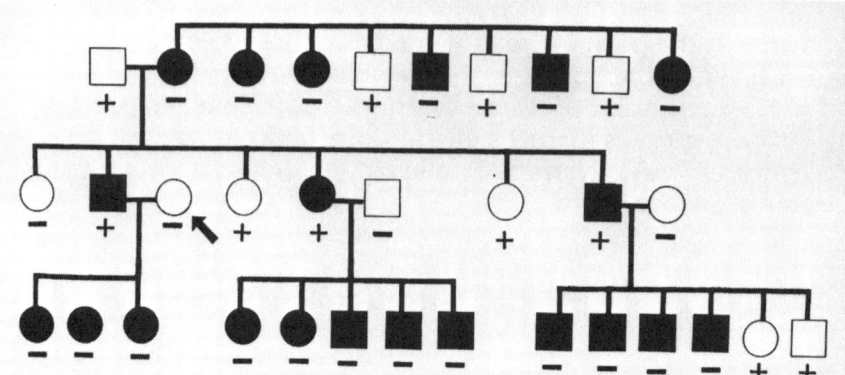

Figure 5-1. Lu9 and Lu^a types in the Mull family. All members of the family are Lu(b+). Black = Lu:9; White = Lu:–9; + = Lu(a+); – = Lu(a–). (Reproduced with permission.[6])

first generation also appeared to be the result of a double backcross mating.

Studies of a random population suggested that Lu9 segregates with Lu^a almost as often as with Lu^b. However, at the time of the random study it was not known that the Mull serum also contained a strong hemagglutinating anti-HLA-B7. This may have skewed the figure of about 2% for the Lu9 antigen. No other examples of anti-Lu9 have been reported.

Lu8 and Lu14

The pairing of Lu8 with Lu14 is a more complicated story. A Caucasian patient with renal failure, Mrs. Hof., had received many transfusions. She produced an antibody that reacted with about 2.4% of random Caucasian red cells. Her Lutheran phenotype consisted of the common antigens in normal doses. When her serum was tested with a large number of cells that expressed known low incidence antigens, the cells of the original Sw(a+) reacted. But additional examples of Sw(a+) cells were negative, and another cell sample, reactive with Mrs. Hof's serum, proved to be negative for Sw^a. Mrs. Hof's antibody was named anti-Lu14.[7]

Adsorption and elution studies, using the original Sw(a+) cells of Mr Swann, confirmed that anti-Sw^a and anti-Lu14 were different antibodies. The Sw(a+) propositus, therefore, had two unusual low frequency red cell antigens. Additional Swann family studies provided more evidence of independence. Mr. Swann's sister typed as Sw(a+) but Lu:–14; both of his children proved to be Sw(a+) but only one was Lu:14.

Mrs. Hof's anti-Lu14 was tested with a large number of red cells negative for high frequency antigens and was found reactive only with the cells of Lu:–8 individuals and their relatives. The antibody gave stronger reactions with Lu:–8 cells than with random Lu:14 cells.

Finding that 14 of 580 random donors were Lu:14, and that only one of the 220 selected Lu(a+b+) cells were Lu:14, suggested linkage disequilibrium of Lu14 with Lu^a. The family of the Lu(a+b+), Lu:14 donor was studied and the Lutheran phenotype and ABH secretor status for this double backcross mating bolstered the probability that Lu14 belonged in the Lutheran system.

A third pair of alleles within the Lutheran system producing Lu8 and Lu14 were, therefore, recognized. A random population of 2000 Caucasians would be apt to have 48 Lu:14 individuals and one Lu:–8 example.[7]

Lu5 and "Singleton"

Enthusiasm for allelic pairs within the expanding Lutheran system abetted the notion that the serum Singleton might be detecting the antithetical antigen for Lu:–5. This was based on the strong reactions obtained with the cells of the Black Lu:–5 proposita. Although the study with the Singleton serum was never published, word of it circulated within the friendly fraternity of blood groupers and the number Lu:10 was reserved for it. This number entered reviews of the Lutheran system and eradication has proved very difficult despite good evidence in ensuing years that it has no relationship with Lu:5 or the Lutheran system.[23]

Additional Cases of the Lutheran-Related Phenotypes

After the first two or three reports of unusual red cell phenotypes, additional cases are seldom published. It is important to have up-dated figures for appraisal of clinical significance and for possible diagnostic and transfusion needs. It is often difficult to gather such information from the far corners of the globe, or even from the nearest blood grouping reference laboratory.

Lu(a–b–) or Lu:–3 Phenotype

Many individuals with the "dominant" form have been found. Only seven people in four families have been reported with the "recessive" phenotype, and five of these had anti-Lu3.

Two other "recessive" Lu(a−b−) names have appeared on rare red cell lists without any serological or lineal information.

Lu:−4 *Phenotype*

There have been no reports since the original case with two compatible siblings.

Lu:−5 *Phenotype*

Another anti-Lu5 was reported, in 1972, in a Black woman with one compatible sibling. The deceased parents were second cousins.[33] Six other individuals with the Lu:−5 phenotype have been studied but not reported. At least five have made anti-Lu5.

Lu:−6 *Phenotype*

A second case of anti-Lu6 with a high titer was reported in 1972.[34] No family study was possible. A third case was found in Denmark with the Lu:−6 phenotype and anti-Lu6, and this woman had a compatible sister.[35] In 1983, a fourth case of anti-Lu6 was reported in an infant with thalassemia major.[36] Eleven other individuals are known to be Lu:−6. At least five, and probably more, made anti-Lu6, but these have not been published.

Lu:−7 *Phenotype*

No further cases have been mentioned.

Lu:−8 *Phenotype*

At least eight more people are known with the phenotype and five or more have made anti-Lu8.

Lu:−9 *Phenotype*

All Lu:−6 individuals are Lu:9.[35] A few heterozygous (Lu:6,9) people have been found. The search for Lu:9 red cells has been hampered by scarcity of the antibody. Only one anti-Lu9 has ever been detected.

Lu:−11 *Phenotype*

No additional cases have been reported, but two other cases are known, both having produced the antibody.

Lu:−12 *Phenotype*

No additional cases have been reported.

Lu:−13 *Phenotype*

Five names have appeared on rare red cell lists and, presumably, some were detected by production of the antibody.

Lu:−14 *Phenotype*

All Lu:−8 individuals are Lu:14. Numerous heterozygous individuals are known. At least 10 more anti-Lu14 samples have been found.

Lu:−16 *Phenotype*

There has been none since the original three cases.

Lu:−17 *Phenotype*

No new cases are known.

Lutheran Linkage and Chromosomal Assignment

Autosomal linkage with a blood group was first reported, in 1951, between Lu^a and the secretor (*Se*) gene.[37] This was initially thought to be a Lutheran-Lewis linkage because *Se* genes determine the expression of Lewis on red cells. It was later shown that the *Le* genes are not closely linked to the *Secretor* or the *Lutheran* locus.[38] However, in recent years, all three (*Lu*, *Le* and *Se*) genes have been assigned to chromosome 19.[8,9]

Chromosome 19 also carries the genes for the complement component C3 and the blood group antigens LW and H. Linkage between Lutheran and myotonic dystrophy was suspected in 1954[39] and established in 1972.[40] The order of the various gene loci assigned to chromosome 19 may be *Le—C3—LW—APO—Lu—Se—H*.

The depression of Au^a in *In(Lu)* individuals initially suggested linkage of Auberger with Lutheran. A large French family, however, showed that these antigens had separate loci.[41]

The inhibitor gene, *In(Lu)*, was shown to be independent of the Lutheran locus and also not linked to *P*.[42] Independence has been shown for the Lutheran inhibitor gene, from *ABO*, *MNSs*, *Rh*, *K*, *Fy*, *Jk*, *Yt* and from the *X* and *Y* loci.[1] The *In(Lu)* gene affects many other antigens, some of which are encoded by genes on the short arm of chromosome 11.[43, 44] These are dealt with in Chapter 6.

Lutheran Serology

Detection

Anti-Lu^a is in short supply largely because it is not sought in donor populations, and if found in patients it is usually accompanied by other antibodies. Red cell screening reagents are not apt to include Lu(a+) cells. Three examples of anti-Lu^a were found in 18,613 blood donors when a deliberate search was made for the antibody.[15] Most laboratories using more than one commercial red cell panel will probably have an Lu(a+) cell at hand and will be able to detect the antibody in patients' sera.

Anti-Lu^b is uncommon rather than really rare in large patient populations. Usually it occurs alone. Most reference laboratories have sufficient frozen samples of Lu(b−) cells to exclude underlying contaminating antibodies. Lu(b−) cells are seldom included in diagnostic red cell panels. A panagglutinin nonreactive with the patient's cells and weaker with Lu(a+b+) and cord cells will suggest anti-Lu^b. The patient would be expected to type as Lu(a+b−). A monoclonal anti-Lu^b will be discussed in Chapter 6.

The high frequency antibodies thought to be within the Lutheran system will be detected only by finding them negative with Lu(a−b−) cells, dominant as well as recessive. Makers of these antibodies usually have common Lutheran phenotypes except for their own rarity. These antibodies are difficult to identify unless null cells are available.

Antigen Strength

Some Lutheran antigens are fragile when stored. Occasionally a red cell sample will appear to be an Lu$_{null}$ cell unless tested when freshly collected. Cells have also been found that seem to have genetically depressed Lutheran antigens and these, too, may be mistaken for Lu$_{null}$ cells. They may be products of another modifying gene at a locus separate from the Lutheran locus or they may be part of the *In(Lu)* complex.

Investigators have found wide variations in antigen strength for both Lu^a and Lu^b. These appear to follow a normal distribution curve. The degree of antigen expression has been found to be genetic in most of the families studied. Exceptionally strong or weak Lu^b cells in red cell diagnostic panels can be helpful for detection of anti-Lu^b if this trait is known.

The third patient recognized as Lu:−6 had a compatible sister whose cells were suitably strong with anti-Lu9 as expected for the Lu:−6,9 phenotype. However, the propositus, whose anti-Lu6 was found after her second pregnancy, reacted very weakly with the only known anti-Lu9 serum. This is still unexplained.[35]

Agglutination Characteristics

The antigen-antibody pattern for Lu^a is often "mixed-field," as though representing two populations of cells. The agglutination has also been described as resembling a "pine tree" in capillary tube tests.[45] Anti-Lu^b seldom produces the tight agglutination seen with Rh or Kell antibodies although the antibodies may have high titers. These agglutination properties may be due to sparse distribution of Lutheran antigens on the red cells.

Test Methods

Many Lutheran antibodies have been found to be saline reactive. This is particularly true of Lu^a antibodies, which usually react better at room temperature. Some rare examples of anti-Lu^a have required AHG serum for detection. Many anti-Lu^b are considered better with AHG testing, but almost all Lutheran antibodies react well with 30% bovine albumin at room temperature in capillary tubes. Dominantly suppressed Lu(a−b−) cells, when compared with Lu(a+b−) cells, often appear slightly grainy in capillary tube tests with anti-Lu^b.

Fetal and Cord Antigen Detection

Although Lu^a has been detected in the blood of a 12-week-old fetus, and Lu^b in two 10-week-old fetal samples, most of those studied have had much weaker antigen expression than adults. This is also true for newborns. Infants who are genetically Lu^aLu^b may have exceedingly weak expression of the antigens and appear to be of null phenotype.[1, 46]

Anti-Lu^a and "Bg"

HLA hemagglutinating antibodies appeared so regularly with Lu^a antibodies that some early investigators were tempted to seek kinship for them. However, they are obviously not linked and there has been no explanation for the frequent companionship of these antibodies. The presence of contaminating HLA antibodies may interfere with accurate testing with some examples of anti-Lu^a.

Rare Cell Needs

The activity records of the National Red Cross rare donor registry show that the need for Lu(b−) units ranks high in the list every year. It would be very helpful to reference laboratories to have Lu(b−) cells included more often in commercial panels.

Clinical Significance of Lutheran and Related Antibodies

Lutheran antibodies can be enormously time consuming for blood bank laboratories although they are rarely clinically significant. There have been a few reports of shortened survival of transfused cells, of elevated levels in macrophage assays and of mild hemolytic disease of the newborn.

Most Lutheran antibodies have been found to be IgM, IgG or mixtures thereof, but some have been said to also be partly IgA. The IgG of anti-Lu^b has been found to be mostly IgG4.[47]

Hemolytic Disease of the Newborn

Lutheran antigens are poorly expressed on cord cells and are therefore unlikely candidates for coating and destruction by maternal Lutheran antibodies. However, there have been four reports of newborns whose direct antiglobulin tests (DAT) were positive, two attributed to anti-Lu^a and two to anti-Lu^b.

The first case, in 1960, was the second baby of a woman who had never been transfused. Her first stillborn baby was too macerated for serological studies. The mother's anti-Lu^b was identified at that time but was not considered responsible for the infant's condition. The titer of the antibody increased to 64 with saline tests and to 256 with antiglobulin tests by the end of her second pregnancy. However, the healthy infant, Lu(a+b+), had a negative DAT. By the sixth day the infant's bilirubin rose to 9.4 mg/dl but there was no anemia and no treatment was necessary. The mother was group A and the child was group AB, so ABO incompatibility could not be definitely ruled out.[48]

The second report, in 1961, of anti-Lu^a in a woman who had never been transfused, resulted in a 2+ DAT in her sixth infant and a weakly positive DAT in her seventh baby. Neither baby needed therapy. The last baby developed a bilirubin of 9.0 mg/dl on the fourth day. The anti-Lu^a was unusual in exhibiting a prozone when titrations were performed four months after the sixth baby was born. At that time the saline titer was 32 at room temperature and 64 at 37 C, but the antiglobulin titer was 1024. During the seventh pregnancy the prozone and the saline reactions disappeared and the AHG titer rose to 4096. The father and three earlier children were Lu(a+b+). Eluates prepared from the cord cells of both involved infants reacted only with Lu(a+) cells.[49]

In 1966 a woman, who had never been transfused, was found to have anti-Lu^b in her serum during her second pregnancy. The baby had a weakly positive DAT. Two days after delivery the bilirubin rose to 7.3 mg/dl. There were no other clinical symptoms. The mother was Rh negative and both babies were Rh positive, but only anti-Lu^b was identified in the mother's serum. It had an antiglobulin titer of 16. The report did not mention any attempts to elute the antibody from the cord cells.[50]

A brief report in 1982 described another example of mild HDN attributed to anti-Lu^a. The mother was group A$_1$, Rh positive, as was the father. No antibodies were detected by routine prenatal screening. The infant had a weakly positive DAT but no antibodies were found in the mother's serum or in the eluate from the cord cells. However, the mother's serum reacted strongly by AHG with the father's red cells. The baby's sample was insufficient for testing of an eluate with the father's cells. A reference laboratory found the mother's serum to contain anti-Lu^a and the father's cells to be Lu(a+). At a later date, the baby's cells were found to be Lu(a+). The infant's bilirubin rose to 13.0 mg/dl the second day and measured 15.8 mg/dl by the fourth day. The course was uneventful after treatment with phototherapy.[51]

An extensive study was reported, in 1982, of an anti-Lu^b in a woman who had never been transfused but who had had several abortions. She was carefully monitored during the next two pregnancies. The DAT was negative in both infants and they had normal hemoglobin and reticulocyte levels, but the antibody was recovered from cord cells with heat elution. After 48 hours there was a rise in bilirubin to 11.4 mg/dl in the first infant and to 12. 5 mg/dl in the second baby. There was no evidence of HDN in either of them. Both babies had the expected Lu(a+b+) phenotype. The mother's antibody was not inactivated by 2-mercaptoethanol (2-ME) and immunoglobulin-class testing suggested that the antibody belonged to the IgG1 subclass. Macrophage assays were performed several times and gave variable results but were usually elevated. The cord red cells were not phagocytized. The AHG titer of the anti-Lu^b ranged from 64 to 256 during this period.[52]

In the large prenatal service of the British Columbia Red Cross three women with anti-Lu14 had Lu:14 infants without evidence of HDN although the Lu14 antigen was well expressed on cord cells.[53]

Lutheran Antibodies in Transfusion

All reported Lu^b antibodies appear to have been immune in origin, but severe hemolytic transfusion reactions have not been caused by Lutheran or Lutheran-related antibodies. However, some of these antibodies have been responsible for shortened survival of transfused red cells and for posttransfusion jaundice.

One of the icteric cases has already been described in the section on the history of anti-Lu^b.[14] Another case of posttransfusion jaundice was reported in 1966. A young male with small bowel disease was found to be Lu(a+b−) with anti-Lu^b in his serum. Several operations for correction of fistulae were complicated by septic and bleeding problems. During one emergency he received four units of Lu(b+) blood. He became icteric with a peak in clinical jaundice 72 hours posttransfusion but suffered no other obvious damage.[54]

Several chromium survival studies of Lu(b+) red cells given to Lu(a+b−) recipients have been published. An early study with a patient whose anti-Lu^b was weakly reactive at 37 C resulted in destruction of 15% of Lu(a+b+) cells in 1 hour but much slower removal of the remaining cells. When the same patient was given a small amount of Lu(a−b+) cells there was rapid removal of 70% of the cells then, again, much slower destruction of the rest of the cells.[55]

In 1977 a patient whose IgG anti-Lu^b had a titer of 256 was given chromium-labeled Lu(a+b+). These had a survival of 94% at 3 hours and 46% at 8 days.[56]

A chromium-survival study was done on a 46-year-old woman, with cancer of the stomach, who had anti-Lu^b. The IgG antibody had a titer of 32 against Lu(a−b+) red cells. The injected chromium-labeled Lu(a−b+) red cells had an 84.4% survival at 60 minutes, but only 8.5% survival at 24 hours.[57] However, it was later suggested that there may have been fairly rapid removal of a small sample, but that a larger amount might have had a better survival record.

A Pakistani baby with thalassemia major, needing frequent transfusions, developed anti-Lu6. Because he was Rh: − 4 and development of anti-c was feared, he was given Rh: − 4, Lu(a−b+) units after chromium studies showed a T_{50} of 26 days with such units. With macrophage assays there was no significant binding of anti-Lu6-coated cells. The patient's antibody was found to be IgG1 and IgG2. The antibody became undetectable despite regular transfusions with Lu(a−b+) units which produced the desired increments in hemoglobin.[36]

Acknowledgments

I am very grateful for the generous help of Dr. Patricia Tippett. Her review of the manuscript corrected sins of omission and commission. If errors remain, they were added after her perusal of the unfinished paper. My thanks also extend to Amy Chung, Joan M. McCreary, Delores A. Mallory, Dr. W. L. Marsh, Marilyn K. Moulds, John J. Moulds, Dr. Marion E. Reid and Dr. G. L. Daniels for information "updating" the Lutheran rare cell and antibody lists.

References

1. Race RR, Sanger R. Blood groups in man. 6th ed. Oxford: Blackwell Scientific Publications, 1975.
2. Cutbush M, Chanerin I. The expected blood-group antibody, anti-Lu^b. Nature 1949;163:580.
3. Crawford MN, Greenwalt TJ, Sasaki T, Tippett P, Sanger, Race RR. The phenotype Lu(a−b−) together with unconventional Kidd groups in one family. Transfusion 1961;1:228-32.
4. Darnborough J, Firth R, Giles CM, Goldsmith KLG, Crawford MN. A "new" antibody anti-Lu^{a}Lu^b and two further examples of the genotype Lu(a−b−). Nature 1963;198:796.
5. Marsh WL. Anti-Lu5, anti-Lu6 and anti-Lu7. Three antibodies defining high frequency antigens related to the Lutheran blood group system. Transfusion 1972;12:27-34.
6. Molthan L, Crawford MN, Marsh WL, Allen FH. Lu9, another new antigen of the Lutheran blood group system. Vox Sang 1973;24:468-71.

7. Judd WJ, Marsh WL, Øyen R, et al. Anti-Lu14: a Lutheran antibody defining the product of an allele at the Lu8 blood group locus. Vox Sang 1977;32:214-9.
8. Gedde-Dahl T Jr, Olaisen B, Teisberg P, Wilhelmy MC, Helland R. The locus for apolipoprotein E (apoE) is close to the Lutheran (Lu) blood group locus on chromosome 19. Hum Genet 1984;67:178-82.
9. Sistonen P. Linkage of the LW blood group with the complement C3 and Lutheran blood group loci. Ann Hum Genet 1984;48:239-42.
10. Callender ST, Race RR. A serological and genetical study of multiple antibodies formed in response to blood transfusion by a patient with lupus erythematosus diffusus. Ann Eugen Lond 1946;13:102-17.
11. Mainwaring UR, Pickles MM. A further case of anti-Lutheran immunization with some studies on its capacity for human sensitization. J Clin Pathol 1948;1:292-4.
12. Lawler SD. The inheritance of the Lutheran blood groups in 47 English families. Ann Eugen Lond 1950;15:255-7.
13. Chown B, Lewis M, Kaita H. The Lutheran blood groups in two Caucasian population samples. Vox Sang 1966;11:108-10.
14. Greenwalt TJ, Sasaki T. The Lutheran blood groups: a second example of anti-Lu^b and three further examples of anti-Lu^a. Blood 1957;12:998-1003.
15. Greenwalt TJ, Sasaki T, Steane EA. The Lutheran blood groups: a progress report with observations on the development of the antigens and characteristics of the antibodies. Transfusion 1967;7:189-200.
16. Tippett P. Serological study of the inheritance of unusual Rh and other blood group phenotypes. PhD thesis, University London, 1963.
17. Crawford MN, Tippett P, Sanger R. The antigens Au^a, i and P_1 of the cells of the dominant type of Lu(a−b−). Vox Sang 1974; 26:283-7.
18. Tippett P. A case of suppressed Lu^a and Lu^b antigens. Vox Sang 1971;20:378-80.
19. Taliano V, Guevin R-M, Tippett P. The genetics of a dominant inhibitor of the Lutheran antigens. Vox Sang 1973;24:42-7.
20. Stanbury A, Francis B. The Lu(a−b−) phenotype: an additional example. Vox Sang 1967;13:441-3.
21. Brown F, Simpson S, Cornwall S, Moore BPL, Øyen R, Marsh WL. The recessive Lu(a−b−) phenotype: a family study. Vox Sang 1974;26:259-64.

22. Myhre B, Thompson M, Anson C, Fishkin B, Carter PK. A further example of the recessive Lu(a−b−) phenotype. Vox Sang 1975;29:66-8.
23. Issitt PD. Applied blood group serology. 3rd ed. Miami: Montgomery Scientific, 1985.
24. Norman PC, Tippett P, Beal RW. An Lu(a−b−) phenotype caused by an X-linked recessive gene. Vox Sang 1986;51:49-52.
25. Shaw MA, Leak MR, Daniels GL, Tippett P. The rare Lutheran blood group phenotype Lu(a−b−): a genetic study. Ann Hum Genet 1984;48:229-37.
26. Udden MM, Umeda M, Hirano Y, Marcus DM. New abnormalities in the morphology, cell surface receptors, and electrolyte metabolism of *In(Lu)* erythrocytes. Blood 1987;1:52-7.
27. Bove JR, Allen FH, Chiewsilp P, Marsh WL, Cleghorn TW. Anti-Lu4: a new antibody related to the Lutheran blood group system. Vox Sang 1971;21:302-10.
28. MacIlroy M, McCreary J, Stroup M. Anti-Lu8, an antibody recognizing another Lutheran-related antigen. Vox Sang 1972;23:455-7.
29. Gralnick MA, Goldfinger D, Hatfield PA, Reid ME, Marsh WL. Anti-Lu11: Another antibody defining a high-frequency antigen related to the Lutheran blood group system. Vox Sang 1974;27:52-6.
30. Sinclair M, Buchanan DI, Tippett P, Sanger R. Another antibody related to the Lutheran blood group system (Much.) Vox Sang 1973;25:156-61.
31. Turner C. Anti-Lu17 (anti-Pataracchia): a new antibody to a high frequency antigen in the Lutheran system. Can J Med Tech 1979;41:43-7.
32. Heddle N, Murphy W. Anti-Lu17. Transfusion 1986;26:306.
33. Bowen AB, Haist AL, Talley LL, Reid ME, Marsh WL. Further examples of the Lutheran Lu(−5) blood type. Vox Sang 1972;23:201-4.
34. Wrobel DM, Moore BPL, Cornwall S, Wray E, Øyen R, Marsh WL. A second example of Lu(−6) in the Lutheran system. Vox Sang 1972;23:205-7.
35. Dybkjaer E, Lylloff K, Tippett P. Weak Lu9 antigen in one Lu:−6 member of a family. Vox Sang 1974;26:94-6.
36. Gibson M, Devenish A, Daniels GL, Contreras M. A transfusion problem in a thalassaemic infant with anti-Lu6 (abstract). Cambridge: British Blood Transfusion Society, 1983.

37. Mohr J. A search for linkage between the Lutheran blood group and other hereditary characters. Acta Pathol Microbiol Scand 1951;28:207-10.
38. Sanger R, Race RR. The Lutheran-secretor linkage in man: support for Mohr's findings. Heredity 1958;12:513-20.
39. Mohr J. A study of linkage in man. Copenhagen, Munksgaard, 1954.
40. Renwick JH, Bundey SE, Ferguson-Smith MA, Izatt MM. Confirmation of linkage of the loci for myotonic dystrophy and ABH secretion. J Med Genet 1971;8:407-16.
41. Salmon C, Rouger P, Liberge G, Streiff F. A family demonstrating the independence between Lutheran and Auberger loci. Rev Fr Transfus Immunohematol 1981;24:339-43.
42. Contreras M, Tippett P. The Lu(a−b−) syndrome and an apparent upset of P_1 inheritance. Vox Sang 1974;27:369-71.
43. Telen MJ, Palker T, Haynes BF. Human erythrocyte antigens:II. The In(Lu) gene regulates expression of an antigen on an 80-kilodalton protein of human erythrocytes. Blood 1984;64:599-606.
44. Francke U, Foellmer BF, Haynes BF. Chromosome mapping of human cell surface molecules: monoclonal antihuman lymphocyte antibodies 4F2, A3D8 and A1G3 define antigens controlled by different regions of chromosome 11. Somatic Cell Mol Genet 1983;9:333-44.
45. Moore BPL, Humphreys P, Lovett-Moseley CA. Serological and immunological methods. The technical manual of the Canadian Red Cross Blood Transfusion Service. 7th ed. Toronto: Canadian Red Cross Society, 1972.
46. Toivanen P, Hironen T. Antigens Duffy, Kell, Kidd, Lutheran and Xg[a] on fetal red cells. Vox Sang. 1973;7:372-6.
47. Mollison PL. Blood transfusion in clinical medicine. 7th ed. Oxford: Blackwell Scientific Publications, 1983.
48. Kissmeyer-Nielsen F. A further example of anti-Lu[b] as a cause of a mild haemolytic disease of the newborn. Vox Sang 1960;5:532-7.
49. Francis BJ, Hatcher DE. Hemolytic disease of the newborn apparently caused by anti-Lu[a]. Transfusion 1961;1:248-50.
50. Scheffer H, Tamaki HT. Anti-Lu[b] and mild hemolytic disease of the newborn. Transfusion 1966;6:497-8.

51. Inderbitzen PE, Windle B. An example of HDN probably due to anti-Lu^a. Transfusion 1982;22:542.
52. Dube VE, Zoes CS. Subclinical hemolytic disease of the newborn associated with IgG anti-Lu^b. Transfusion 1982;22:251-3.
53. Ballem PJ, Stout TD, Battista N, Adatia A, Buskard NA. Significance of anti-Lu14 in hemolytic disease of the newborn. Blood 1987;70(suppl 1):107a.
54. Molthan L, Crawford MN. Three examples of anti-Lu^b and related data. Transfusion 1966;6:584-9.
55. Cutbush M, Mollison PL. Relation between characteristics of blood group antibodies in vitro and associated patterns of red cell destruction in vivo. Br J Haematol 1958;4:115-37.
56. Tilley CA, Crookston MC, Haddad SA, Shumak, KH. Red blood cell survival studies in patients with anti-Ch^a, anti-Yk^a, anti-Ge, and anti-Vel. Transfusion 1977;17:169-72.
57. Peters B, Reid ME, Ellisor SS, Avoy DR. Red cell survival studies of Lu^b incompatible blood in a patient with anti-Lu^b (abstract). Transfusion 1978;18:623.

In: Pierce, SR, and Macpherson, CR, eds.
Blood Group Systems: Duffy, Kidd and Lutheran
Arlington, VA: American Association
of Blood Banks, 1988

6

The Lutheran Blood Group System: Monoclonal Antibodies, Biochemistry and the Effect of In(Lu)

Geoff Daniels, PhD

LUTHERAN IS A COMPLEX blood group system probably comprising at least three closely linked loci, each with two recognized alleles. The "null" phenotype Lu(a−b−) results from one of three different genetic backgrounds: homozygosity for a recessive gene, hemizygosity for an X-linked inhibitor gene or heterozygosity for a dominant inhibitor gene. The dominant gene, called *In(Lu)* (an alternative notation is discussed at the end of the chapter), affects expression of a number of red cell antigens, some of which are known to be produced by genes independent of the *Lutheran* locus (see Chapter 5).

A number of monoclonal antibodies with specificities related to the Lutheran system have proved to be useful tools in the elucidation of the biochemistry of Lutheran and related antigens. Described below is our current perception of the structure of the Lutheran antigens (those antigens produced by genes at the *Lu* complex locus), para-Lutheran antigens [high frequency antigens absent from Lu(a−b−) cells of both dominant and recessive types] and those antigens loosely related to the Lutheran system because of their absence from, or weak expression on, red cells of persons with the *In(Lu)* gene. This knowledge has led to speculation as to the manner by which *In(Lu)* suppresses expression of so many otherwise unrelated structures.

Geoff Daniels, PhD, MRC Blood Group Unit, London, United Kingdom

Monoclonal Antibodies

Monoclonal Anti-Lu^b

Only one monoclonal antibody with specificity for a Lutheran-system antigen has been described, the monoclonal anti-Lu^b BRIC 108 reported by Parsons et al[1] (Table 6-1). BRIC 108 was produced by a hybridoma cloned from a fusion of NS1 mouse myeloma cells and spleen cells from a mouse immunized with Lu(b+) red cells. The antibody agglutinated Lu(a−b+) and Lu(a+b+) cells, but failed to agglutinate Lu(a+b−) cells and Lu(a−b−) cells of dominant, recessive and X-linked types. It also failed to react with Lu:−12 cells, which have a weak Lu^b antigen, but sufficient cells were not available for adsorption/elution tests. Surprisingly, BRIC 108 gave consistently higher titration scores with Lu:14 cells than with Lu:−14 cells.[2] Parsons et al[1] were originally unable to adsorb and elute BRIC 108 from Lu(a+b−) or Lu(a−b−) cells (dominant or recessive). However, using more stringent methods, BRIC 108 was not only eluted from dominant Lu(a−b−) cells,[3,4] as would be expected from studies[5] with human alloanti-Lu^b, but also from recessive Lu(a−b−) cells and from Lu(a+b−) cells.[4,6] Also, using one particular anti-mouse immunoglobulin reagent with BRIC 108, all Lu(b−) cells tested were weakly agglutinated.[6] Therefore, BRIC 108 does not appear to be quite specific for Lu^b, although it does make a good anti-Lu^b reagent when used by agglutination or by the antiglobulin test with an appropriate anti-mouse globulin.

The binding of BRIC 108 to Lu(b+) red cells was inhibited by coating the cells with human anti-Lu^b or anti-Lu3, but not with antibodies unrelated to the Lutheran system.[3] This suggests that both Lu^b and Lu3 determinants are situated in proximity to the BRIC 108 epitope.

BRIC 108 did not react, by immunofluorescence, with mononuclear cells, granulocytes or platelets from a Lu(b+) donor, or with erythroleukemic cell lines K562 and HEL.[1]

BRIC 108 has been used as a tool in the analysis of the structure of the Lu^b antigen and in the estimation of the number of Lu^b binding sites on red cells. These studies are described in the section on biochemistry of Lutheran antigens.

Lutheran-Related Monoclonal Antibodies

A number of monoclonal antibodies have been produced which either fail to react with *In(Lu)* cells [red cells of people with the *In(Lu)* gene], or react less strongly with these cells than

Table 6-1. Monoclonal Antibodies that Show Reduced Reactivity with In(Lu) Red Cells

Specificity	Name	Ig Class	Immunogen*	M_T†
Lu[b1]	BRIC 108 (9W13#)	IgG1	Lu(b+) red cells	85, 78
CDw44 epitope 1[12,33,42,47]	A3D8 (32W2#)	IgM	Malignant Sezary T-cells	80
CDw44 epitope 1[35,42,47]	50E6	IgG2a	Glycoprotein, CLL cells	80
CDw44 epitope 1[32,42,47]	F10.44.2	IgG2a	T lymphocytes	80
CDw44 epitope 2[34,41,42]	A1G3	IgG2	Lymphoma T-cell line	80
CDw44 epitope 3[35,42,47]	50B4	IgG2b	Glycoprotein, CLL cells	80
CDw44 epitope 3[36,42,47]	44D10	IgG1	non-T, non-B ALL line	80
CDw44 epitope 3[47,**]	F10.62.1	IgG1	T lymphocytes	80
CDw44[37]	BRIC 35 (9W11#)	IgG1	Red cells	80
CDw44[38]	OSK-1 (13W1#)	IgG1	Red cells	80
CDw44[43,44,‡]	L21	IgG1	Cord red cells	80
MER2[61]	1D12, 2F7	IgG2a	Small cell carcinoma line	
AnWj[76]	H86	IgG1	ALL T-cell line HSB-2	
Probably AnWj[76]	M447	IgG1	ALL T-cell line MOLT4	

*All cells used for immunizing mice were of human origin
†Apparent molecular weight of major red cell component detected under nonreducing conditions (kD)
#Number used by First International Workshop on Monoclonal Antibodies Against Human Red Blood Cells and Related Antigens
**Fabre J, Lomas C, Tippett P, personal communication
‡Telen M, Marcus D, personal communication

with control cells. These antibodies, which include anti-AnWj, the CDw44 antibodies and anti-MER2, are listed in Table 6-1 and described below in the section on other antigens suppressed by *In(Lu)*. They cannot be considered as Lutheran or para-Lutheran antibodies as they react strongly with recessive Lu(a−b−) cells. Therefore their link with the Lutheran system is phenotypic, since *In(Lu)* also inhibits expression of antigens known to be controlled by genes independent of the *LU* locus (see Chapter 5).

Biochemistry of Lutheran Antigens

The genetics of the Lutheran system, three pairs of alleles at apparently closely linked loci, could suggest a polypeptide chain with three or more sites for amino acid substitution. However, it is also possible that the Lutheran genes encode for transferase enzymes which produce the Lutheran antigens by adding carbohydrate residues to a polypeptide or lipid backbone.

Effect of Heat, Detergents, Enzymes, Reducing Agents and Other Chemicals

Lutheran antigens are thermolabile. Red cells heated to 56 C for 15 minutes are less able to absorb or be agglutinated by Lutheran antibodies (Øyen et al, cited in Marsh[7]). During cold butanol extraction of red cell stroma, Lu^b, Lu3 and Lu4 antigens are found in the aqueous phase, interpreted as suggesting that antigen activity is associated with glycoproteins.[7] Lu^a and Lu^b receptors were almost completely released from red cell membranes by low concentrations of the non-ionic detergent Triton X-100, which specifically renders the integral proteins of red cell membranes soluble.[8] Dahr and Kruger[8] interpreted their chromatographic results as indicating that Lutheran antigens are located on cysteine-containing proteins.

Table 6-2 shows that the Lutheran antigens Lu^a, Lu^b, Lu3, Lu6, Lu8 and Lu14 and the para-Lutheran antigens Lu4, Lu5, Lu12, Lu13 and Lu16 are all destroyed by trypsin treatment and chymotrypsin treatment of the red cells. Papain generally has little effect, with the exception of the "allelic antigens" Lu8 and Lu14. The destruction of Lu8 by papain was previously noted by Poole and Giles.[9] Monoclonal anti-Lu^b did not agglutinate red cells treated with endoglycosidase F/peptidyl *N*-glycosidase F (endo F), which catalyzes the removal

Table 6-2. Reactions of Lutheran, Para-Lutheran and Related Antibodies with Antigen-Positive Red Cells Treated with Various Enzymes and Reducing Agents

Antibodies	No. of Sera	Red Cell Treatments*							
		None	Tryp	Chym	Pap	Sial	AET	DTT 50 mM	DTT 200 mM
Anti-Lu[a]	5	+	0	0	+	+	0	+	0
Lu[b]	18[†]	+	0	0	+	+	0	+	0
Lu3	3	+	0	0	+	+	0	+	0
Lu6	4	+	0	0	+	+	0	+	0
Lu8	2	+	0	0	0	+	0	nt	nt
Lu14	3	+	0	0	0	+	0	+	nt
Lu4	1	+	0	0	+	+	0	+	0
Lu5	1	+	0	0	+	+	0	0	0
Lu12	1	+	0	0	+	+	0	+	0
Lu13	1	+	0	0	+	+	0	+	0
Lu16	1	+	0	0	+	nt	0	+	nt
Au[a]	1	+	0	0	+	+	0	+	0
CDw44	2[§]	+	0	0	0	+	0	0	0
In[b]	2	+	0	0	0	+	0	0	0
AnWj	4**	+	+	+	+	+	+	+	+
MER2	2[‡]	+	0	0	+	+	0	0	0

*Red cells treated as described previously[10,11,92]. Tryp = trypsin, Chym = α-chymotrypsin, Pap = papain, Sial = sialidase, AET = 6% AET (and 8% AET with anti-AnWj); [†]including monoclonal antibody BRIC 108; nt = not tested; [§]BRIC 35 and OSK-1; **including monoclonal antibody H86; [‡]two identical monoclonal antibodies, 1D12 and 2F7.

of N-glycosidically linked oligosaccharides from glycoproteins, although the antibody could be adsorbed and eluted from endo-F-treated cells.[1] Monoclonal anti-Lu^b reacted normally with red cells treated with endo-β-galactosidase.[1]

The effects of sulfhydryl-reducing agents, which break inter- and intrapolypeptide chain disulfide bonds resulting in the unfolding of a protein molecule, are controversial. Advani et al[10] found that 6% 2-aminoethylisothiouronium bromide (AET) did not inactivate Lu^a, Lu^b or Lu3, and Branch et al[11] found no inactivation of Lu^a or Lu^b with a high concentration (200mM) of dithiothreitol (DTT). On the other hand, Parsons et al[1] reported that monoclonal anti-Lu^b would not agglutinate red cells treated with 6% AET or 200mM DTT and that 100mM DTT slightly reduced agglutination. Telen et al[12] found that red cells treated with 8% AET were nonreactive with human anti-Lu^b. Table 6-2 shows that red cells treated with 6% AET or 200mM DTT at pH 8.0 failed to react with all of the Lutheran and para-Lutheran antibodies tested, including a large number of anti-Lu^b.

The results of treating red cells with enzymes and reducing agents suggest that Lutheran antigens are carried on glycoproteins. They further indicate that the presence of intact disulfide bonds and at least one N-glycosidically linked oligosaccharide are important for antigen integrity.

Analysis of Lu^b Antigen by Immunoblotting

Our comprehension of the structure of Lutheran antigens took a step forward following the production of monoclonal anti-Lu^b, a useful tool for probing red cell membrane components separated by electrophoresis.[1] This antibody is described in the section on monoclonal antibodies above.

When immunoblots of red cell membranes, solubilized under nonreducing conditions in the presence of SDS and electrophoresed on 10% or 8% polyacrylamide gels, were probed with the monoclonal anti-Lu^b (BRIC 108), two components of apparent molecular weight 85 kD and 78 kD, respectively, were identified.[1] The 85-kD component was more intensively stained than the 78-kD component. These two components were not apparent when membranes from Lu(a+b−) cells or Lu(a−b−) cells of either recessive or dominant type were used and they were not present in cytoskeleton preparations. No bands were seen when membranes were prepared under reducing conditions—further evidence that antigen expression is dependent on disulfide bonds. Immunoblots from membranes of red cells treated with endo F did not show the 85-kD and 78-kD components, but two new faint bands of molecular weight 73 kD and 66 kD, respectively, were seen. Blots from membranes of cells treated with endo-β-galactosidase appeared no different than those from membranes of untreated cells.

Since endo F catalyzes the cleavage of N-glycosidically linked carbohydrates from glycoproteins, Parsons et al[1] suggested that the 73-kD and 68-kD components seen after treatment with this enzyme represent the 85-kD and 78-kD components, respectively, after loss of one or more N-linked oligosaccharide chains. As mentioned above, BRIC 108 cannot agglutinate endo-F-treated cells, even though it does bind to them to some extent. Thus, N-linked sugars must be important to the expression of the BRIC 108 epitope. Resistance of the BRIC 108-reactive glycoproteins to the action of endo-β-galactosidase suggests that the N-linked structures are not of the poly-N-acetyllactosaminyl type.

Immunoblotting with purified human anti-Lu^a and anti-Lu^b also revealed two components of apparent molecular weight approximately the same as those components recognized by the monoclonal anti-Lu^b (Daniels GL and Khalid G, unpublished observations).

Are Lutheran Antigens Carried on Glycolipids?

All the evidence presented so far leads to the conclusion that Lutheran antigens are carried on glycoproteins. However, Marcus et al[13] reported that Lu^b had been detected in human red cell gangliosides: complex sphingolipids with one or more terminal sialic acid residues. They suggested that Lutheran determinants, like P$_1$ and Ii antigens, contain common glycolipids such as lactoneotetraosylceramide (paragloboside) [Gal(β1→4)GlcNAc(β1→3)Gal(β1→4)Glc-ceramide] or homologous larger structures, or branching structures built on this backbone. Parsons et al[1] point out that this conflicts with their observation that BRIC 108 did not agglutinate trypsin-treated Lu(b+) cells and could not be adsorbed and eluted from trypsin-treated cells. They suggest that the monoclonal antibody may be specific for certain carbohydrate structures only when present in a peptide environments, whereas polyclonal anti-Lu^b may not have this precise requirement for peptide. However, all Lutheran antibodies tested failed to react with trypsin-treated red cells, including all of 18 examples of anti-Lu^b (Table 6-2). Any Lutheran determinants carried on glycolipids must represent a very small proportion of the antigen sites.

The LU gene locus is sited on chromosome 19.[14] Five other "blood group" gene loci are also present on this chromosome: H, SE, LE, LW and OK.[14, 15] H, SE and LE all encode, or control the production of, fucosyltransferases which catalyze the addition of a fucose residue to the carbohydrate chain of a glycoprotein or glycolipid.[16, 17] LW antigens could represent a glycosylated form of the Rh polypeptide and consequently genes at the LW locus may produce the appropriate glycosyltransferase.[18] There is evidence the Ok^a is carried on a series of glycoproteins and thus the Ok^a gene may also encode a glycosyltransferase.[15] Consequently, it is reasonable to speculate that a family of genes is present on chromosome 19, all producing glycosyltransferases responsible for the glycosylation of polypeptides and lipids expressed on the red cell surface and in other tissues.

Estimation of Lu^b Site Density on Red Cells

Merry et al[19] used BRIC 108 monoclonal anti-Lu^b to estimate the number of Lu^b sites on human red cells. The monoclonal antibody was purified and radiolabeled, and the number of molecules of antibody bound per cell was estimated by Scatchard analysis. The results are shown in Table 6-3. Lu(a−b−) cells of the recessive type and trypsin- and pronase-treated cells gave results of between 165 and 280 sites and a figure of some 200 sites was assumed to represent a background of nonspecific antibody binding. X-linked Lu(a−b−) cells gave a result approximately equivalent to background, suggesting either no or very few Lu^b sites. Dominant Lu(a−b−) cells and Lu(a+b−) cells had more sites, although far fewer than most Lu(a+b+) or Lu(a−b+) cells. This is perhaps not surprising, as BRIC 108 has been adsorbed and eluted from cells of both phenotypes.[3, 4, 6] Merry et al[19] point out that adsorption/elution tests had not been done on the Lu(a+b−) cells used in the site number estimation and that some at least could have been genotypically Lu^{a}Lu^b with very weak expression of Lu^b. Lu(a−b+) cells tended to have more Lu^b sites than Lu(a+b+) cells. The main conclusion from this study was that the abundance of Lu^b antigens on red cells is relatively low but shows wide variation,[19] confirming many previous serological studies.

Table 6-3. Estimation of the Number of BRIC 108 Binding Sites on Various Cells

Cell	Molecules of Antibody Bound Per Cell
Trypsin-treated Lu(a−b+)	280
Pronase-treated Lu(a−b+)	210
Lu(a−b−) L.B. (recessive type)	165, 190, 220
Lu(a−b−) Mor. II-6 (X-linked)	260
Lu(a−b−) 3 examples (dominant type)	440–690
Lu(a+b−) 4 examples	320–630
Premature baby (pool)	820
Lu(a+b+) 4 examples*	850–1820
Lu(a−b+) 5 examples*	1640–4070

*Cells of the phenotypes Lu (a−b+) and Lu (a+b+) were selected on the basis of the titration with BRIC 108 or anti-Lu^b as representing the range of serological reaction. (Reprinted with permission from S. Karger AG, Basel.[19])

Other Antigens Suppressed by *In(Lu)*

Described below are serological and biochemical studies on red cell antigens suppressed by the *In(Lu)* gene but which are expressed normally on recessive Lu(a−b−) cells. The serological evidence for the suppression by *In(Lu)* of P_1, i and Au^a is described in Chapter 5.

P_1 and i

Structures of the P_1 and i antigens are well documented. In both antigens the determinants comprise carbohydrate chains. The P_1 oligosaccharide chain is carried on glycosphingolipids with the structure Gal(α1→4)Gal(β1→4)GlcNAc(β1→3)Gal(β1→4)Glc→ceramide. P_1 antigen is produced by the addition of α-galactose to the terminal galactose of lactoneotetraosylceramide (paragloboside), the reaction presumably being catalyzed by an α1→4-galactosyltransferase (for reviews see Marcus et al,[13] Watkins[16] and Issitt.[20(p 209–18)]

Red cell I and i determinants are carried on the ABH-bearing carbohydrate chains of glycolipids and glycoproteins: i, predominantly on the straight chains found in greater abundance on cord red cells than on red cells of most adults; I, on branched chains which are virtually absent from cord red cells (for reviews see Feizi[21] and Issitt[20 (p 192-5)]). Repeating Gal(β1→4)GlcNAc units appear to be required for strong i activity.[21, 22]

Au^a

Virtually nothing is known of the biochemistry of Au^a. In its reactions with enzyme-treated and with AET-treated Au(a+) red cells, anti-Au^a behaves like Lutheran and para-Lutheran antibodies: it reacts with papain-treated cells but not with trypsin-, chymotrypsin- or AET-treated cells (Table 6-2).

Cs^a, Yk^a, Kn^a, McC^a and Sl^a

From a series of family studies, Daniels et al[23] showed that cells with the dominant Lu(a−b−) phenotype are more often weak for Cs^a, Yk^a, Kn^a, McC^a and Sl^a than are those from the general population, although the effect is not so dramatic as that for P$_1$, i and Au^a. Like Au^a, virtually nothing is known regarding the biochemistry of these antigens. These antigens are mostly sensitive to treatment of the red cells with trypsin or α-chymotrypsin (Daniels GL, unpublished observations), but—with the possible exception of Yk^a, for which there is some disagreement[24, 25]—insensitive to ficin and papain treatment[24, 26-29] (Daniels GL, unpublished observations). Moulds and Moulds[30] reported that red cells treated with 6% AET were inactive with anti-Yk^a, anti-Kn^a and anti-McC^a, although Marsh et al[31] found that cells treated in this way could still adsorb these antibodies.

The CDw44 Glycoprotein

A3D8 and Related Monoclonal Antibodies

Numerous monoclonal antibodies,[12, 32-38] that react with many different human cell types—including T-cells, granulocytes, brain cells, epithelial cell lines and red blood cells—detect epitopes on a common glycoprotein. Antibodies that react with this glycoprotein have been assigned to a cluster CDw44 by the Third International Workshop on Human Leukocyte Differentiation Antigens.[39]

The first of the CDw44 antibodies reported to be detecting a determinant suppressed by In(Lu) was A3D8.[12] Telen et al[12, 40] found that when red cells were analyzed by flow cytofluorography, A3D8 reacted with all red cells, including cord cells and Lu(a−b−) cells of dominant, recessive and X-linked types. However, four examples of dominant Lu(a−b−) cells all showed markedly reduced levels of binding.[12] Since then a number of similar antibodies that demonstrate reduced levels of binding to In(Lu) cells have been described[34, 37, 38, 41, 42] (Table 6-1). Some agglutinate cells of common Lutheran type but not In(Lu) cells,[3, 37, 41] although they do react with In(Lu) cells by an antiglobulin test. With some CDw44 antibodies, the effect of In(Lu) on the strength of reactions is not apparent by ordinary serological methods. No reduction in titer with In(Lu) cells was seen with the definitive CDw44 antibody F10.44.2 by an antiglobulin test (Lomas G, Tippett P, personal communication), although immunofluorescence-activated flow cytometry demonstrated a 75% reduction in binding to In(Lu) cells.[42] Binding of two of these antibodies (BRIC 35, OSK-1) with Lu(a−b+) cells was not "blocked" by coating the cells with human anti-Lu^b or anti-Lu3.[3]

Another CDw44 monoclonal antibody, L21, was used at a dilution of 1/2000 to screen for Lu(a−b−) in blood donors of the Houston metropolitan region.[43, 44] Of 42,000 tested, eight had red cells that either failed to react or reacted weakly with the antibody; all were Lu(a−b−).

A3D8 antigen was detected in serum. Serum of Lu(b+) people reduced red cell binding by the A3D8 antibody by 67%, whereas serum from a dominant Lu(a−b−) individual reduced binding by only 33%.[12]

Structure of the CDw44 Glycoprotein

Immunological reactivity of the CDw44 glycoprotein is destroyed, or partially destroyed, by treatment of the red cells with the enzymes trypsin, α-chymotrypsin, pronase, papain or bromelase and with the reducing agents AET and DTT[3, 12, 33, 37, 42, 45, 46] (Table 6-2), and therefore depends on intact inter- and/or intrachain disulfide bonding. It is not affected by sialidase treatment of the red cells.

A major component of molecular weight 80 kD (called[34] p80) was revealed by immunoprecipitation of solubilized red-cell membranes with CDw44 antibodies followed by SDS-PAGE under reducing or nonreducing conditions,[33, 41] or by immunoblotting with CDw44 antibodies of red cell membranes electrophoresed on a 10% polyacrylamide gel under nonreducing conditions.[33, 37, 41] Under reducing conditions no band was present on immunoblots. Immunoprecipitation and immu-

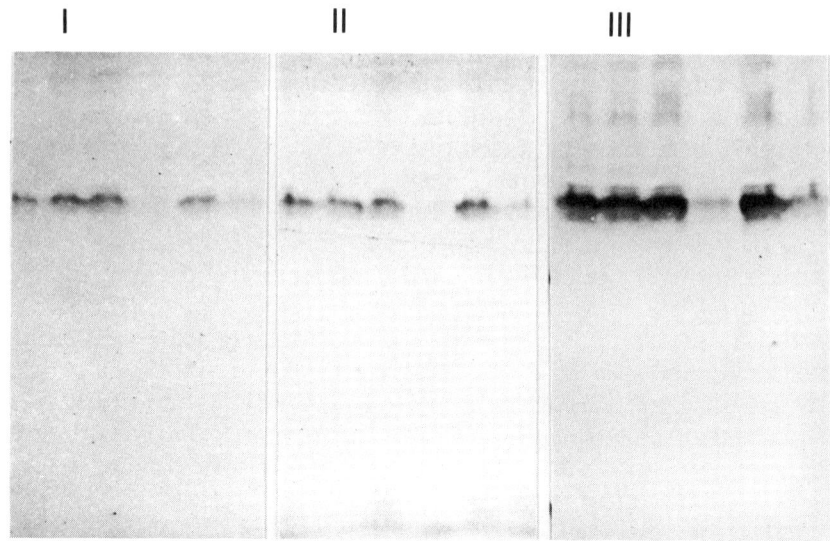

a b c d e f a b c d e f a b c d e f

Figure 6-1. Immunoblots of red cell membranes electrophoresed under nonreducing conditions on a 10% polyacrylamide gel and probed with the CDw44 antibodies BRIC 35 (I) OSK-1 (II) and A3D8 (III). A. Lu(a−b+) membranes. B. Lu(a+b−) membranes. C through F. membranes from *In(Lu)* family: c. Lu(a−b+) sister, D. Lu(a−b−) propositus, E. Lu(a−b+) mother, F. Lu(a−b−) father.

noblotting of dominant Lu(a−b−) membranes revealed only a trace of p80,[33, 37, 41] (Fig 6-1) whereas recessive and X-linked Lu(a−b−) cells had normal, or even slightly enhanced, expression of p80.[6, 40] When immunoblotting followed SDS-PAGE on an 8% gel the apparent molecular weight of p80 had shifted to 85 kD, a familiar phenomenon for glycoproteins.[37]

Immunoblotting of endo-F-treated red cells, which revealed a substantial reduction in molecular weight of the p80 component,[37, 42] and the binding of p80 to concanavalin A and lentil lectins,[42] demonstrated that the molecule is a glycoprotein that contains at least one N-glycosidically linked oligosaccharide chain. Lack of apparent alteration of p80 in endo-β-galactosidase-treated cells suggests that the molecule does not contain extensive polylactosaminyl groups. The glycoprotein does not contain a substantial number of O-glycosidically linked sugars, as immunoblotting of sialidase-treated cells or Tn cells (in which the O-linked sialotetrasaccharides, normally found on red cell sialoglycoproteins, are modified) also revealed little or no reduction in the molecular weight of p80.[6, 37]

Using a variety of antibodies to the CDw44 glycoprotein, Letarte[47] and Telen et al[42] showed that these antibodies define at least three epitopes on the glycoprotein molecule (Table 6-1). Antibodies that detect all three epitopes showed substantially reduced binding to *In(Lu)* red cells compared with Lu(b+) cells.[42]

CDw44 Glycoprotein on Cells Other than Red Cells

The CDw44 glycoprotein, originally called[32] the human brain-granulocyte-T-lymphocyte antigen, is a ubiquitous structure present on cells from a variety of tissues. As well as being detected on circulating B and T lymphocytes, granulocytes and mononuclear cells[12, 32, 37] and a variety of normal and leukemic cell lineages,[12, 35-37] CDw44 glycoprotein is present in brain, heart, liver, thymus, breast, colon epithelium, kidney and lung and on squamous epithelial cells of skin, cornea and conjunctiva.[12, 32, 34, 36, 48-54] Telen et al[12, 41] found that *In(Lu)* individuals had increased numbers of lymphocytes that fail to react with the monoclonal antibodies A3D8 and A1G3 compared with those of control donors, although those lymphocytes that expressed the antigen appeared to express it normally. Monocytes from Lu(b+) donors exhibited uniformly strong reactivity with the antibody whereas monocytes from the *In(Lu)* donors showed two populations of cells, one subset strongly antigen-positive and another antigen-negative or only weakly positive.

The function of the CDw44 glycoprotein on red cells is unknown. In the thymus medulla it may play a role in normal maturation of thymocytes.[32, 34, 36] In brain it is virtually restricted to the white matter,[50, 51, 53] but in elderly people and victims of multiple sclerosis it is detected in low concentrations in gray matter and in significantly higher concentrations than usual in white matter.[51, 52] The antigen may be expressed on fibrous astrocytes,[50, 53] which form a supporting framework for nerve cells and may serve as phagocytes, removing degenerating neuronal material.[54, 55] In disease, astrocytes also fill spaces vacated by dead neurons. Cells carrying the CDw44 determinant in the kidney may have similar supporting or phagocytic functions.[54]

The Gene that Encodes the CDw44 Structure

Goodfellow et al,[56] by testing the original antibody in CDw44 (F10.44.2) against a panel of somatic cell hybrids, showed that the determinant recognized by that antibody was encoded by a gene on human chromosome 11. This was later confirmed, using a different antibody (A3D8), and localized to the short arm of chromosome 11.[57]

In^a and In^b

The low-frequency red cell antigen In^a and the high-frequency antigen In^b were recently shown by Spring et al[37] to be carried on the CDw44 glycoprotein. Subsequently, expression of In^b was found[37] to be suppressed by *In(Lu)*. In^a and In^b are probably the products of alleles,[58] but this has not been formally proven. Their presence on the same glycoprotein is additional evidence for allelic status.

In^a and In^b both detect protease- and DTT-sensitive red cell antigens[8, 37, 58-60] (Table 6-2). Immunoblotting after electrophoresis of antigen-positive membranes under nonreducing conditions on a 10% gel, showed that purified human anti-In^a and anti-In^b both detect a component of apparent molecular weight of around 80 kD: no 80-kD component was detected in membranes from In(a−) and In(b−) cells, respectively.[37] A band of markedly reduced intensity was seen with membranes from *In(Lu)* cells blotted with anti-In^b. As with blots probed by the monoclonal antibody BRIC 35, the In^b-reactive component gave a higher molecular weight on 8% gels.

Anti-In^b (and the CDw44 monoclonal antibody BRIC 35) bound to glycoprotein isolated from human leukocytes with F.10.44.2, the original CDw44 antibody.[37] Also, substance immunoprecipitated from human red cell membranes by BRIC 35 reacted with anti-In^b on an immunoblot, proof that the In^b determinant is carried on the CDw44 glycoprotein.[37]

MER2

MER2 is a red cell polymorphism defined by two monoclonal antibodies, 1D12 and 2F7 (Table 6-1): 92% of English blood donors are MER2+ and 8% MER2−.[61] Strength of expression of MER2 varies. Anti-MER2 monoclonal antibodies reacted with Lu(a−b−) cells of dominant, recessive and X-linked types. However, when the antibodies were titrated with red cells from members of a large three-generation family in which *In(Lu)* was segregating, the following scores were obtained[62]: nine Lu(a−b−) members varied from 0-15 with a mean of 6; 12 Lu(a−b+) members varied from 12-21 with a mean of 16. This suggests that *In(Lu)* suppresses the expression of MER2.

Very little is known regarding the structure of the MER2 antigen. MER2 antigen on red cells is sensitive to trypsin and α-chymotrypsin, but not to papain, ficin or sialidase. It is also sensitive to the reducing agents AET and DTT[61] (Table 6-2). Thus MER2 is probably carried on a glycoprotein, the reactivity being dependent on the presence of intact disulfide bonds.

The gene coding for MER2, like the gene coding for CDw44 glycoprotein, is on the short arm of chromosome 11.[61] They are sited at different regions on that chromosome, however.[63]

AnWj

Anton

The first mention of anti-Anton was by Boorman and Tippett (cited in Race and Sanger[64 (p 274–5)]) in 1972 and Daniels[65] described a second example in 1980. Both antibodies failed to react with dominant Lu(a−b−) cells and cord cells, but Lu(a−b−) cells of the recessive type were not available for testing. Both antibodies fixed complement and reacted with papain- and with trypsin-treated cells.[65] The notation Lu15 was set aside for Anton but was shown to be inappropriate when Poole and Giles[9] showed that five examples of anti-Anton reacted with recessive Lu(a−b−) cells. They also pointed out that, unlike the Lutheran and para-Lutheran antigens, Anton antigen was not destroyed by trypsin treatment. A number of other Anton− individuals with anti-Anton have been identified since, yet there is still no evidence that the Anton− phenotype is inherited: at least eight sibs of Anton− propositi have been tested[9,66] and all were Anton+. It therefore appears likely that Anton−, other than in Lu(a−b−) persons, is an acquired character.

Wj

Anti-Wj, an autoantibody, was first reported in 1983 by Marsh et al[67] after a preliminary report[68] at the American Associations of Blood Banks' Annual Meeting 2 years previously. Another autoantibody reported[69] at the same meeting was probably also anti-Wj.[70] The original anti-Wj was found in the serum of an Lu(a−b+) patient with systemic lupus erythematosus and slight anemia, as well as in eluates from her red cells.[67,68] The antibody reacted with red cells from 415 random donors and three recessive Lu(a−b−) individuals, but failed to react with 14 examples of the dominant type and with cord cells, although some binding of Lu(a−b−) of anti-Wj to dominant Lu(a−b−) cells could be demonstrated by adsorption and elution. Anti-Wj did not appear to be clinically significant: transfusion of the patient with one unit of least-incompatible blood apparently had no harmful effect. Anti-Wj was not considered[67] to be responsible for the patient's slight anemia.

Anton and Wj Are the Same

In 1985 Poole and Giles[71] suggested that even though anti-Anton were allo-reactive antibodies and anti-Wj was an autoantibody, they might be detecting the same determinant. Subsequently, Mannessier et al[72] described a Hodgkin's disease patient with a temporary acquired loss of Wj antigen. Red cells of the patient were negative with four examples of anti-Wj autoantibodies and were also negative with anti-Anton. Serum of the patient contained an antibody described[72] as allo-anti-Wj. At remission, six months later, the antibody had disappeared and the patient's cells were Wj+ and Anton+. Anti-Anton and anti-Wj have since been confirmed as having the same specificity (Poole J, personal communication).

In 1986 the International Society of Blood Transfusion Working Party for Terminology for Red Cell Surface Antigens[73] gave the new name AnWj to both Anton and Wj. AnWj is now included among the antigens of high frequency, and numbered 900030. Lu15 (005015) is now obsolete.

Development of AnWj Antigen

In a study of red cells from 36 infants, Poole and Van Alphen[74] showed that the age at which conversion from AnWj− to AnWj+ takes place varies from infant to infant but occurs between the ages of 3 days and 46 days and requires less than 1 day to complete. This rapid or "all-or-nothing" phenomenon is unexpected as the red cells in the circulation are not all produced at the same time and no evidence could be found for a conversion factor in the serum.[74] However, whatever causes the change from AnWj− to AnWj+ in infants is presumably reversible on rare occasions, since the adult AnWj− phenotype has not been shown to be inherited and can be transient. The transient AnWj− phenotype with concurrent presence of anti-AnWj has been recognized in a couple of patients[72,75] and in a healthy individual (Poole J, cited in Poole and Van Alphen[74]). The original AnWj− individual remained AnWj− for many years (Boorman KE and Tippett P, personal communication).

Monoclonal Anti-AnWj

Knowles et al[76] described two monoclonal antibodies (H86 and M447) produced from a fusion of NS1 cells and spleen cells from mice immunized with human T-cell lines derived from patients with acute lymphocytic leukemia (Table 6-1). These antibodies reacted with red cells by the antiglobulin test, using selected anti-mouse globulin, strength of reaction being enhanced by papain or trypsin treatment of the cells. They failed to react with cord cells and with Lu(a−b−) cells of the dominant type, but did react with recessive Lu(a−b−) cells and were later shown to react with Lu(a−b−) cells of the X-linked type.[76, 77]

Knowles et al[76] and Poole and Giles[9] remarked that H86 and M447 behaved like the antibodies now called anti-AnWj. Later, Mannessier et al[72] found that red cells of a transiently AnWj− patient were negative with H86 while they were AnWj−, but reacted with H86 when they became AnWj+. H86 has since been shown to fail to react with two more samples of AnWj− cells with normal Lutheran antigens and to react weakly with an AnWj-weak sample (Poole J, personal communication; Daniels GL, unpublished observations). Since M447 appears to have the same specificity, it is probably also anti-AnWj.

AnWj as a Receptor for Haemophilus Influenzae

Although the bacterium *Haemophilus influenzae* is a commensal of the throat of most healthy people, it may also cause respiratory tract infections and, more seriously, is a major cause of bacterial meningitis in young children. Strains of *H. influenzae* that express fimbriae (short, threadlike processes attached to the cell walls) agglutinate red cells. The fimbriae are believed to be involved in adherence to nasopharyngeal epithelial cells.[78]

Van Alphen et al[79] showed that while fimbriae-bearing strains of *H. influenzae* isolated from patients with invasive disease and respiratory tract infections agglutinated most red cell samples from adults—including recessive Lu(a−b−) cells—they failed to agglutinate cord cells, In(Lu) cells and cells of two Lu(a−b+) AnWj− persons. Anti-AnWj inhibited agglutination of AnWj+ red cells by the bacteria. However, *H. influenzae* bound to buccal epithelial cells from six neonates as strongly as to epithelial cells of adults, even though the bacteria failed to agglutinate the red cells of five of the six babies.[80] Also, adherence of *H. influenzae* to epithelial cells was not inhibited by anti-AnWj and the bacteria adhered to epithelial cells of an AnWj− individual.[80] Thus, although the AnWj antigen appears to be the structure on red cells bound by *H. influenzae* fimbriae, it is not the receptor for adherence to epithelial cells and consequently is probably not relevant to infection.

Antilymphocyte Globulin

Purified antilymphocyte globulin (ALG), produced in horses by the injection of human lymphocytes or cultured human lymphoblasts, is used in the prevention of immunological rejection of renal and other organ grafts following transplantation.[81, 82] One complication of this treatment is that the patients' red cells give a positive direct antiglobulin test (DAT) which may create difficulties in pretransfusion crossmatching.[83-86] This positive DAT may become apparent as soon as the first day after the start of treatment with ALG. It is caused by anti-horse antibodies in the anti-human globulin reagent. These contaminating antibodies react with horse anti-human lymphocyte globulin which binds to human red cells as well as human lymphocytes.[87] This anti-horse fraction can be removed by absorbing the antiglobulin reagent with red cells coated with ALG.[83, 84, 87] ALG and serum of patients who receive ALG treatment reacted with human red cells by direct agglutination and by the antiglobulin test.

Anderson et al[85] noticed that eluates from red cells of patients with a positive DAT resulting from ALG treatment failed to react with Lu(a−b−) cells. Neat ALG behaved as a panagglutinin with a titer of about 204,800 with cells of common Lutheran type but only 6400 with Lu(a−b−) cells. Unfortunately the type of Lu(a−b−) was not specified. However, Postoway and Garratty[87] showed that diluted ALG that failed to react with In(Lu) cells reacted strongly with Lu(a−b−) cells of the recessive type. Thus equine ALG is detecting one of the many red cell antigens suppressed by the *In(Lu)* gene.

Concanavalin A Lectin Receptor

Udden et al[44] found that red cells of all five *In(Lu)* individuals from two families demonstrated reduced agglutination with concanavalin A lectin compared with cells of the other family members. Because membrane protein band 3 is the major concanavalin A binding protein, this reduction in binding was interpreted[44] as suggesting an abnormality in glycosylation of band 3 in *In(Lu)* cells.

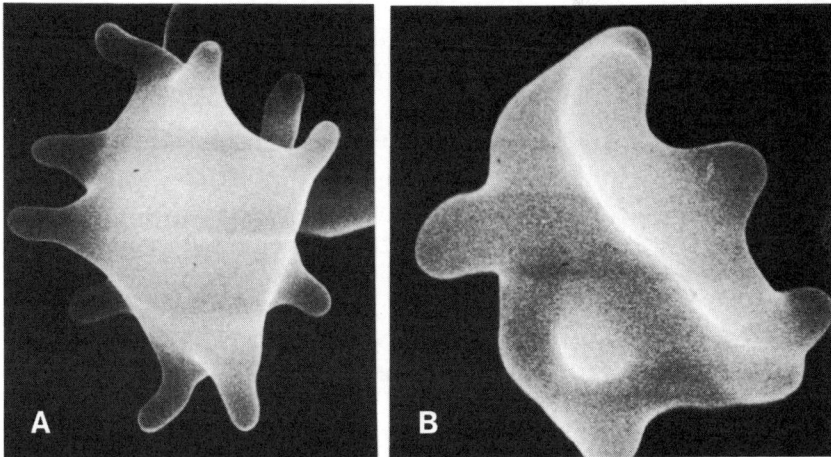

Figure 6-2. Scanning electron micrographs of washed red cells from an *In(Lu)* Lu(a−b−) individual showing an acanthocyte (A) and a bizarre poikilocyte (B). (Reprinted with permission.[44])

The Effect of the Dominant Inhibitor Gene *In(Lu)*

Abnormal Morphology of *In(Lu)* Cells

The effect of *In(Lu)* on red cell shape varies in different families, and even within a family. Udden et al[44] observed the morphology of red cells of members of two *In(Lu)* families. In one family acanthocytes were present among the red cells of both *In(Lu)* members, and acanthocytes and other bizarrely shaped red cells were seen when glutaraldehyde-fixed *In(Lu)* cells were viewed by scanning electron microscopy (Fig 6-2). In the other family the *In(Lu)* propositus had mild poikilocytosis and the occasional acanthocyte but no morphological abnormalities of the red cells of the *In(Lu)* father and aunt of the propositus were observed.

None of the family members with common Lutheran phenotype, from either of the families, demonstrated any red cell morphological abnormalities. Both propositi were healthy. Absence of anemia or reticulocytosis in both families suggests that the abnormal red cell morphology is not associated with significant hemolysis. Morphological examinations of the cells of the original *In(Lu)* proposita suggested that they are normal when freshly bled, but become abnormal during storage at a rate greater than that for cells of common Lutheran type (Crawford MN, personal communication). Abnormal red cell morphology in some persons with an *In(Lu)* gene is pertinent to the observation by Spring et al[37] that at least a proportion of the CDw44 glycoprotein remains associated with the red cell cytoskeleton after extraction with 10% Triton X-100.

Abnormal Electrolyte Metabolism of *In(Lu)* Cells

Osomotic fragility of *In(Lu)* cells is normal.[44] However, incubation of *In(Lu)* cells in plasma for 24 hours at 37 C resulted in significant resistance to osmotic lysis compared with cells of common Lutheran type, in which the osmotic fragility increases.[44] Although both *In(Lu)* and control cells demonstrated similar concentrations of Na^+ and K^+ ions before incubation, during incubation *In(Lu)* cells—but not control cells—lost K^+ and, to a lesser extent, gained Na^+ ions. This reduction in total cation content in *In(Lu)* red cells could explain their relative resistance to osmotic lysis.[44] Crawford noticed a greater degree of hemolysis of the cells from the *In(Lu)* members of her family than of cells from other members, during storage at 4 C in modified Alsever's solution (Crawford MN, personal communication).

How Does the *In(Lu)* Gene Suppress Expression of so Many Red Cell Surface Antigens?

Dominant genes that cause suppression of expression of a gene at another locus are unusual in human genetics; such an inhibitor gene that affects blood group genes at several different loci is so far unique. Consequently models do not exist on which to base an explanation for the mechanism of *In(Lu)*.

The biochemical analyses described above show that Lu^b, i and the CDw44 determinants (including In^a and In^b) are all carried on glycoproteins. The effect of proteases and reducing agents on Au^a, Cs^a, Yk^a, Kn^a, McC^a, Sl^a and MER2 are not incompatible with their being glycoprotein also. P_1 is carried on a glycolipid, as is i and possibly Lu^b. It is, therefore, not inconceivable that the *In(Lu)* gene effects glycosylation of a variety of glycoproteins and glycolipids.

Marcus et al[13] proposed that the *In(Lu)* phenotype may result from the presence of a glycosyltransferase which adds an extraneous sugar to a backbone structure shared by Lutheran antigens, P_1, i and Au^a. Udden et al[44] added that decreased expression of concanavalin A receptor suggests abnormality of glycosylation of band 3, further evidence for *In(Lu)* being responsible for aberrant glycosylation of a common carbohydrate sequence present in many glycoproteins

Table 6-4. Proposed Notations for Dominant Inhibitor of Lutheran and Other Cell Surface Antigens

	Taliano et al[89]	Marsh et al[91]
Locus	*In(Lu)*	*SYN-1*
Rare "dominant inhibitor" gene	*In(Lu)*	*SYN-1 B*
Common "recessive" gene	*In(Lu)*	*SYN-1 A*

and some glycolipids. Also, the presence of the *In(Lu)*-sensitive CDw44 determinants on several different cell lineages—red cells, monocytes and lymphocytes—is more consistent with a carbohydrate than a peptide determinant.[44] However, the molecular weight of the CDw44 glycoprotein of *In(Lu)* cells does not appear to be different from that of red cells of common Lutheran type, evidence against the addition of carbohydrate molecules by the *In(Lu)* product.[37, 42]

An alternative effect of the *In(Lu)* gene, suggested by Shaw and Tippett,[88] is to alter membrane conformation indirectly, thus reducing the quantity of antigen presented to the antibody or impeding antigen binding. They also propose the possibility that some antigens are suppressed by *In(Lu)* directly as a result of abnormal glycosylation; and that others are suppressed indirectly by changes in membrane conformation resulting from abnormal glycosylation of unrelated structures.

Is the Name *In(Lu)* Still Appropriate?

In(Lu) was the name given by Taliano et al[89] for the rare, unlinked suppressor of the Lutheran antigens, dominant in effect over the common gene *In(Lu)* (Table 6-4). At that time they were aware[90] that *In(Lu)* probably inhibited expression of Au^a, a blood group antigen genetically independent of Lutheran, but not of the variety of other antigens regulated by the *In(Lu)* gene. The discovery that *In(Lu)* also inhibited expression of P_1 and i antigens led Race and Sanger[64] to say, "This new finding has, of course, made the notation *In(Lu)* less appropriate, and no doubt in time someone will think of a better." Marsh et al[91] subsequently came up with an alternative notation; whether or not it is better is open to debate.

Marsh et al[91] argue that the name *In(Lu)* implies that all antigens affected are closely related to the Lutheran system. They propose that the *In(Lu)* locus be renamed *SYN: SYN-1 B*, being the rare dominant gene which prevents normal biosynthesis of a number of red cell determinants; *SYN-1 A* the common allele which, in the absence of *SYN-1 B*, permits normal biosynthesis (Table 6-4). A possible third allele, *SYN-1 C*, may be responsible for the Lu(w) phenotype. The name "SYN" is derived from "synthesis."

Although Shaw and Tippett[88] agree that the notation "*In(Lu)*" is outmoded, they also believe that a new name implying that the *In(Lu)* gene modifies antigen synthesis is premature while the mechanism of the effect of this gene remains undetermined. They argue, as described above, that *In(Lu)* may affect the expression of some antigens indirectly by altering membrane conformation and that "a modification of antigen synthesis" would not accurately describe such a mechanism. Shaw and Tippett[88] suggest that the naming of unlinked inhibitor genes be referred to the International Society of Blood Transfusion Working Party on the Terminology of Red Cell Antigens.

In view of the rate at which the biochemical understanding of the structure of antigens affected by *In(Lu)* continues to increase, it is unlikely to be long before the mechanism of the gene interaction is understood. Surely the renaming of the gene could wait until then, in order to avoid the danger of introducing another inappropriate notation.

References

1. Parsons SF, Mallinson G, Judson PA, Anstee DJ, Tanner MJA, Daniels GL. Evidence that the Lu^b blood group antigen is located on red cell membrane glycoproteins of 85 and 78 kD. Transfusion 1987;27:61-3.
2. Zelinski T, Kaita H, Lewis M. Preliminary serological studies of 4 monoclonal antibody samples with "Lutheran" specificities. Rev Fr Transfus Immunohematol (in press).
3. Daniels G. Lutheran-related antibodies. Rev Fr Transfus Immunohematol (in press).
4. Telen M. Report on group 8 antibodies. Rev Fr Transfus Immunohematol (in press).
5. Stanbury A, Francis B. The Lu(a−b−) phenotype: an additional example. Vox Sang 1967;13:441-3.
6. Judson PA, Spring FA, Parsons SF, Anstee DJ, Mallinson G. Report on group 8 (Lutheran) antibodies. Rev Fr Transfus Immunohematol (in press).

7. Marsh WL. Recent developments relating to the Duffy and Lutheran blood groups. In: A seminar on recent advances in immunohematology. Washington, DC: American Association of Blood Banks, 1973:101-19.
8. Dahr W, Kruger J. Solubilization of various blood group antigens by Triton X-100. Proceedings of the 10th International Congress of the Society for Forensic Haemogenetics, Munich. 1983:141-6.
9. Poole J, Giles CM. Observations on the Anton antigen and antibody. Vox Sang 1982;43:220-2.
10. Advani H, Zamor J, Judd WJ, Johnson CL, Marsh WL. Inactivation of Kell blood group antigens by 2-aminoethylisothiouronium bromide. Br J Haematol 1982; 51:107-15.
11. Branch DR, Muensch HA, Sy Siok Hian AL, Petz LD. Disulphide bonds are a requirement for Kell and Cartwright (Yt^a) blood group antigen integrity. Br J Haematol 1983;54:573-8.
12. Telen MJ, Eisenbarth GS, Haynes BF. Human erythrocyte antigens. Regulation of expression of a novel erythrocyte surface antigen by the inhibitor Lutheran *In(Lu)* gene. J Clin Invest 1983;71:1878-86.
13. Marcus DM, Kundu SK, Suzuki A. The P blood group system: recent progress in immunochemistry and genetics. Semin Hematol 1981;18:63-71.
14. Tippett P. Immunogenetics: blood group systems. In: Hackel E, ed. Human genetics 1984: a look at the last ten years—and the next ten. Arlington, VA: American Association of Blood Banks, 1985:1-16.
15. Williams BP, Daniels GL, Pym B, et al. Biochemical and genetical analysis of the Ok^a blood group antigen. Immunogenetics 1988;27:322-9.
16. Watkins WM. Biochemistry and genetics of the ABO, Lewis, and P blood group systems. In: Harris H, Hirschhorn K, eds. Advances in human genetics. New York: Plenum, 1980:1-136.
17. Oriol R, Le Pendu J, Mollicone R. Genetics of ABO, H, Lewis, X and related antigens. Vox Sang 1986;51:161-71.
18. Mallinson G, Martin PG, Anstee DJ, et al. Identification and partial characterization of the human erythrocyte membrane component(s) which express the antigens of the LW blood group system. Biochem J 1986;234:649-52.

19. Merry AH, Gardner B, Parsons SF, Anstee DJ. Estimation of the number of binding sites for a murine monoclonal anti-Lu^b on human erythrocytes. Vox Sang 1987;53:57-60.
20. Issitt PD. Applied blood group serology, 3rd ed. Miami: Montgomery Scientific, 1985.
21. Feizi T. The blood group Ii system: a carbohydrate antigen system defined by naturally monoclonal or oligoclonal autoantibodies of man. Immunol Commun 1981;10:127-56.
22. Gooi HC, Veyrières A, Alais J, Scudder P, Hounsell EF, Feizi T. Further studies of the specificities of monoclonal anti-i and anti-I antibodies using chemically synthesized, linear oligosaccharides of the poly-N-acetyllactosamine series. Mol Immunol 1984;21:1099-104.
23. Daniels GL, Shaw MA, Lomas CG, Leak MR, Tippett P. The effect of *In(Lu)* on some high-frequency antigens. Transfusion 1986;26:171-2.
24. Molthan L. The serology of the York-Cost-McCoy-Knops red blood cell system. Am J Med Tech 1983;49:49-56.
25. Molthan L, Giles CM. A new antigen, Yk^a (York), and its relationship to Cs^a (Cost). Vox Sang 1975;29:145-53.
26. Giles CM, Huth MC, Wilson TE, Lewis HBM, Grove GEB. Three examples of a new antibody, anti-Cs^a, which reacts with 98% of red cell samples. Vox Sang 1965;10:405-15.
27. Molthan L, Moulds J. A new antigen, McC^a (McCoy), and its relationship to Kn^a (Knops). Transfusion 1978;18:566-8.
28. Lacey P, Laird-Fryer B, Block U, Lair J, Guilbeau L, Moulds JJ. A new high incidence blood group factor, Sl^a, and its hypothetical allele (abstract). Transfusion 1980;20:632.
29. Molthan L. The new McCoy antigens, McC^c and McC^d (abstract). Transfusion 1980;20:622.
30. Moulds JJ, Moulds MK. Inactivation of Kell blood group antigens by 2-aminoethylisothiouronium bromide. Transfusion 1983;23:274-5.
31. Marsh WL, Johnson CL, Mueller KA. AET-treated red cells. Transfusion 1983;23:275.
32. Dalchau R, Kirkley J, Fabre JW. Monoclonal antibody to a human brain-granulocyte-T-lymphocyte antigen probably homologous to the W 3/13 antigen of the rat. Eur J Immunol 1980;10:745-9.
33. Telen MJ, Palker TJ, Haynes BF. Human erythrocyte antigens: II. The *In(Lu)* gene regulates expression of an

antigen on an 80-kilodalton protein of human erythrocytes. Blood 1984; 64:599-606.
34. Haynes BF, Harden EA, Telen MJ, et al. Differentiation of human T lymphocytes. 1. Acquisition of a novel human cell surface protein (p80) during normal intrathymic T cell maturation. J Immunol 1983;131:1195-200.
35. Letarte M, Iturbe S, Quackenbush EJ. A glycoprotein of molecular weight 85,000 on human cells of B-lineage: detection with a family of monoclonal antibodies. Mol Immunol 1985;22:113-24.
36. Quackenbush EJ, Letarte M. Identification of several cell surface proteins of non-T, non-B acute lymphoblastic leukemia by using monoclonal antibodies. J Immunol 1985;134:1276-85.
37. Spring FA, Dalchau R, Daniels GL, et al. The In^a and In^b blood group antigens are located on a glycoprotein of M_r 80,000 (the CDw44 glycoprotein) whose expression is influenced by the *In(Lu)* gene. Immunology 1988; 64:37-43.
38. Okubo Y, Seno T, Yamano H, Yamaguchi H. Test results of four monoclonal antibodies against markers of the Lutheran system. Rev Fr Transfus Immunohematol (in press).
39. Cobbold S, Hale G, Waldmann H. Summary of studies performed on the non-lineage, LFA-1 family, and leucocyte common antigen panel of antibodies. In: McMichael AJ, et al. Leucocyte typing III: white cell differentiation antigens. Oxford, UK: Oxford University Press, 1987:788–803.
40. Telen MJ, Green A. Expression of *In(Lu)*-related p80 antigens by autosomal and X-linked recessive Lu(a−b−) erythrocytes (abstract). Transfusion 1987;27:547.
41. Telen MJ, Shehata H, Haynes BF. Human medullary thymocyte p80 antigen and *In(Lu)*-related p80 antigen reside on the same protein. Hum Immunol 1986;17:311-24.
42. Telen MJ, Rogers I, Letarte M. Further characterization of erythrocyte p80 and the membrane protein defect of *In(Lu)* Lu(a−b−) erythrocytes. Blood 1987;70:1475-81.
43. Schultz M, Fortes P, Miller A, Leu L. Use of a monoclonal antibody in determining the frequency of the *In(Lu)* gene (abstract). Transfusion 1985;25:449.
44. Udden MM, Umeda M, Hirano Y, Marcus DM. New abnormalities in the morphology, cell surface receptors, and electrolyte metabolism of *In(Lu)* erythrocytes. Blood 1987;69:52-7.

45. Telen MJ, Letarte M. The membrane glycoprotein defect of *In(Lu)* Lu(a−b−) erythrocytes (abstract). Transfusion 1986;26:574.
46. Poole J, Merry AH, Campbell EJ. Serological and immunochemical characterization of "Lutheran-related" monoclonal antibodies 9W11, 9W13, 13W1 and 32W2. Rev Fr Transfus Immunohematol (in press).
47. Letarte M. Human p85 glycoprotein bears three distinct epitopes defined by several monoclonal antibodies. Mol Immunol 1986;23:639-44.
48. Daar AS, Fabre JW. Demonstration with monoclonal antibodies of an unusual mononuclear cell infiltrate and loss of normal epithelial membrane antigens in human breast carcinomas. Lancet 1981;1:434-8.
49. Daar AS, Fabre JW. The membrane antigens of human colorectal cancer cells: demonstration with monoclonal antibodies of heterogeneity within and between tumours and of anomolous expression of HLA-DR. Eur J Cancer Clin Oncol 1983;19:209-20.
50. McKenzie JL, Dalchau R, Fabre JW. Biochemical characterization and localization in brain of a human brain-leucocyte membrane glycoprotein recognized by a monoclonal antibody. J Neurochem 1982;39:1461-6.
51. Cruz TF, Quackenbush EJ, Letarte M, Moscarello MA. Effects of development and aging on the concentration of a human brain antigen. Neurosci Lett 1985;59:253-7.
52. Cruz TF, Quackenbush EJ, Letarte M, Moscarello MA. Elevated levels of a glycoprotein antigen (p-80) in gray and white matter of brain from victims of multiple sclerosis. Neurochem Res 1986;11:877-89.
53. Quackenbush EJ, Cruz TF, Moscarello MA, Letarte M. Identification of three antigens in human brain associated with similar antigens on human leukaemic cells. Biochem J 1985;225:291-9.
54. Quackenbush EJ, Gougos A, Baumal R, Letarte M. Differential localization within human kidney of five membrane proteins expressed on acute lymphoblastic leukemia cells. J Immunol 1986;136:118-24.
55. Snell RS. Clinical neuroanatomy for medical students, 2nd ed. Boston, MA: Little, Brown and Co, 1987.
56. Goodfellow PN, Banting G, Wiles MV, et al. The gene MIC4, which controls expression of the antigen defined by monoclonal antibody F10.44.2, is on human chromosome 11. Eur J Immunol 1982;12:659-63.

57. Francke U, Foellmer BE, Haynes BF. Chromosome mapping of human cell surface molecules: monoclonal antihuman lymphocyte antibodies 4F2, A3D8, and A1G3 define antigens controlled by different regions of chromosome 11. Somatic Cell Mol Genet 1983;9:333-44.
58. Giles CM. Antithetical relationship of anti-In^a with the Salis antibody. Vox Sang 1975;29:73-6.
59. Badakere SS, Parab BB, Bhatia HM. Further observations on the In^a (Indian) antigen in Indian populations. Vox Sang 1974;26:400-3.
60. Bhatia HM, Badakere SS, Mokashi SA, Parab BB. Studies on the blood group antigen In^a. Immunol Commun 1980;9:203-15.
61. Daniels GL, Tippett P, Palmer DK, Miller YE, Geyer D, Jones C. MER2: a red cell polymorphism defined by monoclonal antibodies. Vox Sang 1987;52:107-10.
62. Tippett P. Contribution of monoclonal antibodies to understanding one new and some old blood group systems. In: Garratty G, ed. Red cell antigens and antibodies. Arlington, VA: American Association of Blood Banks, 1986:84-6.
63. Kazazian HH, Junien C. Report of the committee on the genetic constitution of chromosomes 10, 11 and 12. Human Gene Mapping 9 (1987): Ninth International Workshop on Human Gene Mapping. Cytogenet Cell Genet 1987;46:188-212.
64. Race RR, Sanger R. Blood groups in man. Oxford, UK: Blackwell, 1975.
65. Daniels GL. Blood group antigens of high frequency: a serological and genetical study (thesis). London, UK: University of London, 1980.
66. Harrison CR, Heinz R, Chaudhuri TK. Clinical management of a patient with anti-Anton (abstract). Transfusion 1985;25:463.
67. Marsh WL, Brown PJ, DiNapoli J, et al. Anti-Wj: an autoantibody that defines a high-incidence antigen modified by the *In(Lu)* gene. Transfusion 1983;23:128-30.
68. Brown P, Wood M, Beck ML, et al. An auto-antibody that defines a public antigen suppressed by the *In(Lu)* gene (abstract). Transfusion 1981;21:632-3.
69. Fitzsimmons J, Caggiano V. Autoantibody to a high frequency Lutheran antigen associated with immune hemolytic anemia and a hemolytic transfusion episode (abstract). Transfusion 1981;21;612.

70. Ward JM, Caggiano V. Clarification. Transfusion 1983;23:174.
71. Poole J, Giles C. Anton and Wj, are they related? Transfusion 1985;25:443.
72. Mannessier L, Rouger P, Johnson CL, Mueller KA, Marsh WL. Acquired loss of red-cell Wj antigen in a patient with Hodgkin's disease. Vox Sang 1986;50:240-4.
73. The Working Party on Terminology for Red Cell Surface Antigens. International Society of Blood Transfusion Newsletter 1987;34:5.
74. Poole J, Van Alphen L. *Haemophilus influenzae* receptor and the AnWj antigen. Transfusion 1988 (in press).
75. Harris T, Steiert S, Marsh WL, Berman LB. A Wj-negative patient with anti-Wj. Transfusion 1986;26:117.
76. Knowles RW, Bai Y, Lomas C, Green C, Tippett P. Two monoclonal antibodies detecting high frequency antigens absent from red cells of the dominant type of Lu(a−b−) Lu:−3. J Immunogenet 1982;9:353-7.
77. Norman PC, Tippett P, Beal RW. An Lu(a−b−) phenotype caused by an X-linked recessive gene. Vox Sang 1986;51:49-52.
78. Turk DC. The pathogenicity of *Haemophilus influenzae*. J Med Microbiol 1984;18:1-16.
79. Van Alphen L, Poole J, Overbeeke M. The Anton blood group antigen is the erythrocyte receptor for *Haemophilus influenzae*. FEMS Microbiol Letts 1986;37:69-71.
80. Van Alphen L, Poole J, Geelen L, Zanen HC. The erythrocyte and epithelial cell receptors for *Haemophilus influenzae* are expressed independently. Infect Immun 1987;55:2355-8.
81. Najarian JS, Simmons RL, Condie RM, et al. Seven years' experience with antilymphoblast globulin for renal transplantation from cadaver donors. Ann Surg 1976;184:352-68.
82. Sabiston DC. Textbook of surgery, the biological basis of modern surgical practice, 13th ed. Philadelphia: WB Saunders, 1986.
83. Swanson JL, Mann EW, Condie RM, Simmons RL, McCullough JJ. Resolution of crossmatching problems associated with patients receiving anti-lymphocyte globulin (abstract). Transfusion 1982;22:415.
84. Lapinid IM, Steib MD, Noto TA. Positive direct antiglobulin tests with anti-lymphocyte globulin. Am J Clin Pathol 1984;81:514-7.

85. Anderson HJ, Aubuchon JP, Draper EK, Ballas SK. Transfusion problems in renal allograft recipients. Antilymphocyte globulin showing Lutheran system specificity. Transfusion 1985;25:47-50.
86. Ballas SK, Draper EK, Dignam CM. Pre-transfusion testing problems caused by anti-lymphocyte globulin and their solution. Transfusion 1985;25:254-6.
87. Postoway N, Garratty G. Mechanisms causing positive antiglobulin tests subsequent to anti-lymphocyte globulin (ALG) administration (abstract). Transfusion 1984;24:427.
88. Shaw MA, Tippett P. Proposed new notation for *In(Lu)* modifying gene—another view. Transfusion 1985;25:170-1.
89. Taliano V, Guèvin RM, Tippett P. The genetics of a dominant inhibitor of the Lutheran antigens. Vox Sang 1973;24:42-7.
90. Tippett P. Serological study of the inheritance of unusual Rh and other blood group phenotypes (thesis). London, UK: University of London, 1963.
91. Marsh WL, Johnson CL, Mueller KA. Proposed new notation for the *In(Lu)* modifying gene. Transfusion 1984;24:371-2.
92. Daniels G. Kell-related antibodies. Rev Fr Transfus Immunohematol, (in press).

Index

(Page numbers in italics indicate tables or figures.)

A

A3D8, 128-129
AIHA. *See* Hemolytic anemia, autoimmune
Anti-AnWj, monoclonal, 135
Anti-Fs, 8-9
Anti-Fy3, 5-6
Anti-Fy4, 6-7
Anti-Fy5, 7-8
Anti-Fy6, 9
Anti-Fy^a, 2
    dosage, 2
    HDN, 13
Anti-Fy^b, 2
    dosage, 2
Anti-Lu^a, 109-110
Anti-Lu^b, monoclonal, 120
Antilymphocyte globulin (ALG), Lu(a−b−), and, 136
Anton, 133, 134
AnWj, 133-136
    antigen development, 134
    H. influenzae receptor, 135-136
Asians
    Fy, 13-*14*
    Fy genes and genotypes, *16*
Australians
    Fy, *14*, 15
    Fy genes and genotypes, *16*

B

Blacks
    Fy(a−b−), 1, *11*, 13-*14*-15, 18, *19*
    Fy genes and genotypes, *16*
    Kidd, 54
    malaria, 33, 43
BRIC, 108
    glycolipids, and, 125-126
    immunoblotting, 124-125
    site density on red cells, 126-*127*

C

Cad red cells, 45
Caucasians. *See* Whites
CDw44 glycoprotein, 128-132
    gene that encodes structure, 131-132
    other than red cells, and, 131
    structure, 129-*130*-131
Concanavalin A lectin receptor, In(Lu) and, 136
Cs^a, 128

D

Drugs, Kidd antibodies and, 73-74
Duffy antibodies
    characteristics, *10*
    clinical significance, 12-13
    red cell reactions, *11*
Duffy antigens, 4
    development, fetal red cells, 15
    distribution, 13-*14*-15
    inheritance, 17-18, *19*
    location, 27
    phenotypes, 13-*14*-15
    primates, nonhuman, 15, 17
    synthesis, 17-18
Duffy blood group system, 1-52
    biochemistry, 27-*28*-30
    malaria, 31-43
    nomenclature, 9, 12
    notation, *12*
    See also Fy

F

Fy
    alloimmunization, 2-3
    autoimmunization, 3
    frequency, 3-4
    gene localization and linkage, 17
    genes and genotypes, *16*
    immunogenicity, 3-4
    See also Duffy
Fy3, 5-6, 30
    Plasmodium receptor, 43
Fy4, 6-7
Fy5, 7-8
    Plasmodium receptor, 43
Fy5, 7-8
    Plasmodium receptor, 43
Fy6, 9, 30

Plasmodium receptor, 43
Fy^a, 29-30
   merozoite proteins, 42
   See also Fy
Fy^b, merozoite proteins, 42
   See also Fy
Fy^x, 5

H

HDN. *See* Hemolytic disease of the newborn
Hemolytic anemia, autoimmune (AIHA), Kidd antibodies, 73
Hemolytic disease of the newborn
   Duffy antibodies, 13
   Kidd antibodies, 61-62
   Lutheran antibodies, 110-112
Hemolytic transfusion reaction (HTR), Kidd antibodies, 59, 60

I

i, 127-128
In^a, 132
In^b, 132
Indians, FY, *11*
In(Lu), 96-97, *99*
     antigens suppressed by, 127-139
     concanavalin A lectin receptor, and, 136
     electrolyte metabolism, 138
     inhibitor gene, 137-140
     monoclonal antibodies, and, 120-*121*-122
   notation, *139*-140
   red cell morphology, *137*-138
   red cell surface antigen suppression, 138-139

K

K, 3-4
Kidd antibodies, 59-66
   drug-related, 73-*74*
   HDN, 61-62
   HTR, 59, 60
   in vitro, 62-63
   LISS-related, 74-77-78
   paraben-associated, 76-77
   test methods, *58*, 63-64
Kidd antigens, 57-*58*-59
   alteration, 59
   biochemistry, 78, *79*
   genetic models, 84-86
   immune response to, 59
   location, 77-78
   number, 77-78
   transport, 81-84, *85*
   urea lysis phenomenon, 78-*80*-81, *82*
Kidd autoantibodies, 64-*65*-66
Kidd blood group system, 53-92
   chromosome assignment, 57
   disease association, 86-88
   genetics, 53-*54*-*55*-*56*-57
Kn^a, 128

L

LISS, Kidd antibodies and, 74-77-78
Lu5, 105
Lu6, 103-104
Lu8, 104-105
Lu9, 103-*104*
Lu14, 104-105
Lu:−3, 105-106
Lu:−4, 106
Lu:−5, 106
Lu:−6, 106
Lu:−7, 106
Lu:−8, 106
Lu:−9, 106
Lu:−11, 106
Lu:−12, 107
Lu:−13, 107
Lu:−14, 107
Lu:−16, 107
Lu:−17, 107
Lu^a, 94-95
Lu(a−b−), 105-106
   ALG, and, 136
Lu^b, 95-96
   site density on red cells, 126-*127*
Lu^b antigen, immunoblotting, 124-125
LuLu, 97-98, *99*
Lu$_{null}$, 96-*99*-100
   frequency, 99-100
Lu, X-linked, 98-*99*
Lutheran antibodies
   clinical significance, 110-113
   transfusion, 112-113
   See also Lutheran monoclonal antibodies; Lutheran-related antibodies
Lutheran antigens
   biochemistry, 122-*123-127*
   enzymes, and, 122-*123*-124

fetal and cord cells, detection, 109
glycolipids, and, 125-126
heat, and, 122
reducing agents, and, *123*, 124
strength, 108-109
See also Anti-Lu
Lutheran blood group system, 93-147
allelic pairs, 103-107
biochemistry, 119
linkage and chromosomal assignment, 107-108
phenotypes, common, 94-96
serology, 108-110
Lutheran monoclonal antibodies, 120-*121*-122
In(Lu) and, 120-*121*-122
Lutheran-related antibodies, 100-103
clinical significance, 110-113
See also Lutheran antibodies; Lutheran monoclonal antibodies
Lutheran-related antigens, 100-103
Lutheran serology
detection, 108
rare cell needs, 110
test methods, 109

M

Malaria, 31-46
Duffy, and, 31-43
infection hypothesis, 35-37-42
vaccine, 46-47
See also *Plasmodium* spp.
McC^a, 128
McLeod phenotype, 86
MER2, 132-133
Merozoites
P. falciparum-red cell interactions, 41
P. knowlesi-red cell interactions, 38-*39*-40-41
proteins, 41-42
M^{k}M^k red cells, 45
MN SGP, 44, 45
Monoclonal antibodies
AnWj, 135
BRIC 108, 124-27
Lu, 120-*121*-122
Lu-related, 120, 122

P

Paraben, Kidd antibodies, 76-77
P$_1$, 127-128
Plasmodium
life cycle, 31-*32*-33
receptor sites, 42-43
P. falciparum, 35
merozoite proteins, 42
sialic-acid-dependent sites, 43-44
sialic-acid-independent sites, 46
Wr(a+b−) phenotype, 45-46
P. knowlesi
Duffy antigens, in vitro, 33-34, *35*
infection hypothesis, 35-*37*-38
merozoite proteins, 42
merozoite-red cell interactions, 38-*39*-40
receptor sites, 42
P. vivax
Duffy antigens, in vitro, 34-*35*
receptor sites, 42
Platelets, Fy, 4
Protein, merozoites, 41-42

S

Sialic acid and receptor sites, *P. falciparum*, 43-44, 46
Singleton, 105
Sl^a, 128
Ss SGP, 44, 45
Staph protein A, Fy, 29
SYN-1, *139*, 140

T-U

Tn red cells, 44-45
Transfusion, Lu antibodies, 112-113
Urea lysis phenomenon, Kidd antigens, 78-*80*-81, *82*

W-Y

Whites
Fy, 3, *11*, 13-*14*-15, 18, *19*
Fy genes and genotypes, *16*
malaria, 43
Wj, 133-134
Wr(a+b−) phenotype, 45-46
Yk^a, 128